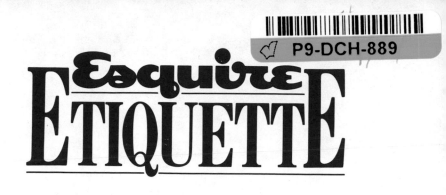

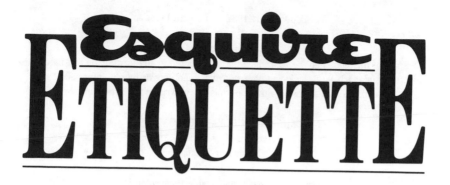

ETIQUETTE

The Modern Man's Guide to Good Form

Glen Waggoner & Kathleen Moloney
—— With the Editors of Esquire ——

An Esquire Press Book

COLLIER BOOKS
Macmillan Publishing Company
New York
Collier Macmillan Publishers
London

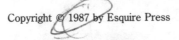
MACMILLAN PUBLISHING COMPANY
866 Third Avenue, New York, N.Y. 10022
Collier Macmillan Canada, Inc.

Library of Congress Cataloging-in-Publication Data

Waggoner, Glen.
  Esquire etiquette.

  "An Esquire Press book."
  1. Etiquette for men.   I. Moloney, Kathleen.
II. Title.
BJ1855.W34   1987   395'.142   87-9301
ISBN 0-02-026240-X

Macmillan books are available at special discounts for bulk purchases for sales promotions, premiums, fund-raising, or educational use. For details, contact:

Special Sales Director
Macmillan Publishing Company
866 Third Avenue
New York, N.Y. 10022

10 9 8 7 6 5

PRINTED IN THE UNITED STATES OF AMERICA

Esquire Etiquette: The Modern Man's Guide to Good Form is also available in a hardcover edition from Macmillan Publishing Company.

CONTENTS

FOREWORD

SINCE ITS FOUNDING in 1933, *Esquire* magazine has spoken authoritatively on matters of importance to men. Personal style, modern fiction, current affairs, contemporary culture—in virtually every area that men care about, *Esquire* has helped define standards of taste and quality.

That includes manners. Not the sort of manners that govern "how things should be done to please delicate ladies tsk-tsking over the teacups in their Victorian bowers," wrote *Esquire* editors in a preface to the 1959 edition of *The New Esquire Etiquette*, first published in 1953. "Instead," they continued, in explanation of what the new edition was about, "it tells you how things are done, by practical men who know their way around in these high-pressure days."

Times change, and so do manners. You will not find here detailed instructions on when and how to tip your hat, for the obvious reason that you do not wear one. Even so, the underlying philosophy that informed *Esquire Etiquette* a generation ago is alive and well in the volume you now hold in your hands. Idiosyncratic and often surprising in its focus, this book is, above all, rooted in a commitment to practicality.

"How things are done by practical men" does not, it must be made clear at the outset, mean how *everything* is done. Do not be misled by the "A to Z" format of this book: It is not, nor was it intended to be, utterly comprehensive in its consideration of rules of etiquette. Heft a copy of a recent edition of Emily Post and you'll spot the difference at once. For specific advice on such matters as how to address the Pope and what sort of present to buy a couple on their twelfth wedding anniversary, we recommend that you consult Ms. (or would she prefer Miss?) Post. (We also heartily recommend the works of Judith Martin, who amply deserves the title "Miss Manners." She brings to the task of monitoring and guiding social conduct a marvelous blend of wit, style, and good sense.)

In a special foreword written for the 1959 edition, *Esquire* founder Arnold Gingrich noted that *Esquire Etiquette* "has been the surprise success of all the books ever issued under the aegis of The Magazine for Men." Gingrich admitted that he and his colleagues were somewhat mystified by its success. After all, he wrote, "this book deals with manners, an always scarce commodity and one that has for a long time appeared to be in diminishing demand. Worse, it deals with Manners for Men. Who needs it? Or would admit it if he did?" The best explanation that Gingrich could come up with to explain *Esquire Etiquette*'s reception was that "word got around somehow that here was one etiquette book that could be read for fun."

We want *this* etiquette book to be read for fun, too. After all, some of the so-called Rules of Etiquette are, if you look at them up close, good *only* for a laugh. Yet most of the books written about them are no fun at all. In a rapidly changing world, we think it is important to bring to any discussion of social conduct a healthy skepticism, a strong sense of one's own values, and a generous sense of humor.

We invite you to share ours.

—Lee Eisenberg
Editor-in-Chief
Esquire, 1987

ACKNOWLEDGMENTS

WE WISH TO EXTEND special thanks to our editor, John Glusman, and to our agent, Dominick Abel.

We are also grateful to Priscilla Flood, who, while director of Esquire Press, launched this project; to Diane Lilly and Tom Robotham, who helped keep it on course; and to Anita Leclerc, who sets the tone and standards as editor of *Esquire*'s "Man At His Best"—where parts of this book first saw light—that we seek to equal here.

Finally, we appreciate the support and encouragement of Betsy Carter, Phillip Moffitt, and Sharon McIntosh, and of Lee Eisenberg, who was willing to take a chance.

G.W. and K.M.

DEDICATION

This book is dedicated to the memory of Marguerite and Henry Waggoner, who taught their son that "ma'am" and "sir" were the most important words in the language after "please" and "thank you"; and to Wini and Ed Moloney, who taught their daughter never to chew gum in public and always to stand when a priest enters the room.

ANSWERING MACHINES

When the first steam locomotive chugged through the English countryside in the 1820s, otherwise sane people labeled it the handiwork of the devil and shrieked that the end of civilization was nigh. So have other harbingers of progress been greeted throughout history. Which brings us to the answering machine.

Some people today still grumble or become suddenly confused when a machine answers, and too many slam down the receiver without leaving a message. These are the same people, mind you, who are perfectly comfortable with internal combustion and the miracle of flight. Well, it's time to grow up. Answering machines are at least as common as blenders in the modern household, and twice as useful. Since they're here to stay, we'd all best learn to appreciate—and use—them.

Start with the premise that having an answering machine is a convenience to your friends, and that cooperating with theirs is a courtesy to them. Even if you're an electronic Luddite who thinks television should have been strangled at birth, remember your reason for calling in the first place: to get in touch with the person who's not in just now, but who was thoughtful enough to employ a device that will register your attempt.

Courtesy and common sense require that you leave a clear, uncomplicated message on a friend's machine. The day and time of your call will be helpful, even if not requested. Don't complain about having to talk to a machine. Don't *talk* to the machine ("Hi, Allison's Machine. Good to hear your voice. Tell your owner I called, will you?"). And don't hang up without saying a word unless your intention is to exasperate rather than communicate.

On your own machine, keep your message short and direct. Don't apologize for not being home, don't promise to call back "as soon as I possibly can," and resist the temptation to be creative. No invented personae. And positively no anthropomorphism ("This is Norton, Peter's cat. If you'll purr a message after the beep tone, I'll lick his face and make sure he gets it when he returns. *Meow*").

A precious few imaginative souls give great answering machine, but more often a frustrated caller must endure embarrassing soliloquies, off-key songs, and badly scripted playlets just for the privilege of leaving a name and number. *Beep tone* is redundant, and *tone* is more precise than *beep,* so say *tone.* If you absolutely cannot resist an occasional exception to good answering-machine form, go whole hog: Mount a real production number, complete with sound effects—even a light show if you can manage it.

The perfect message? "Hello, you have reached 976-1313. If you'd care to leave a message, you may do so after the tone." That says it all.

APOLOGIES

Did Ryan say it to Ali, or vice versa? Who remembers? But we do remember, "Love means never having to say you're sorry." And gosh, it still makes us gag.

"I'm sorry," along with "Please" and "Thank you" (see THANK YOU) are among the most valuable words in the English language, and will be until human beings figure out how to be perfect. We all screw up, hurt those close to us, and act like jerks far too frequently to feel smug about facing life stripped of the ability to beg forgiveness. And assuming that a loved one should forgive you without your even acknowledging your misdeed merely adds arrogance to the list of your transgressions.

Apologies, to be effective, should be kept simple, to the point, and infrequent.

Simple. An elaborate *mea culpa,* complete with histrionics and painstaking detail, deflects attention away from the ill you've done and beams it back on you. In *apologia* circles, this is known as having your cake and eating it. As the transgressor, you must heal another's wounds and beg forgiveness for having inflicted them, not make someone else feel sorry for being justifiably angry with you in the first place.

To the point. Before saying "I'm sorry," make sure you have it clear in your mind just what you're sorry for. "I'm sorry you got mad" and "I'm sorry for being so thoughtless" are *not* the same thing. Try to look at what you said or did from the other person's perspective so you can see how to redress your wrongdoing. (Just because you have a skin thicker than a rhinoceros's doesn't mean you can say any old thing with impunity.) If your 25-words-or-less definition of what it is you did that requires an apology doesn't jibe with the injured party's notion, all you've done by saying you're sorry is take a giant step sideways.

Infrequent. The two little words under discussion work better, of course, the less they're used. This means two things:

being a good guy more of the time (and we know you have it in you) and not feeling the obligation to apologize for every little mistake. For goodness' sake, "Love means not having to say you're sorry" for *everything*.

AUTOMOBILES

Like it or not, in virtually every place in America besides New York City, you are what you drive. (In New York you are where you spend your summer weekends, but that's another story.) And like most things you own that reflect your sense of style and taste, the best choice in cars has nothing to do with trends or expense. It's not necessary to have a really expensive or flashy set of wheels. In fact, driving a status-oriented dream machine that you obviously can't afford can mark you as a most insecure sort of fellow indeed. So don't even consider taking out a loan against your inheritance to put your hands on that bottle-green Porsche. And impressing women with your horsepower ranks right up there with taking ads in the Personals columns and wearing a sandwich board with your salary and phone number on it.

No, to thine own self—and thine own wallet—be true. There's nothing wrong with sensible transportation, and you needn't turn your Saab into a sexmobile. A five-year-old MG that you have fixed up yourself or a VW Rabbit with a good sound-system may be perfect, depending on your needs. Just keep it clean inside and out, and don't get carried away with the decor. Religious medals, fuzzy dice, zebra seat covers, and bouncing hula girls are out.

While real men *do* change their own tires and know which end goes where when using jumper cables, they don't find it necessary to spend the better part of their weekends with their feet sticking out from under the car.

Unless you're 18 and/or still unsure of your manhood, you don't need to be to told that speed kills and that you shouldn't drive after drinking. This is more than a matter of etiquette and consideration of others, of course—it's a matter of law.

Now a few words about automobile manners. When getting out of a car, try to open the door for a woman (always going around the front of the car), but unless she missed the 1960s and

1970s completely, she'll probably be on the sidewalk before you get there. If you're out with another couple, it's standard procedure to ride with your date—even if you've got some important baseball stats to discuss with your buddy.

If it's your car, you drive, but if it's hers, don't feel emasculated if she wants you to sit shotgun instead. Do offer to drive, but take it like a man if she declines. Don't press her for an explanation. And when you're on the road and sorely tempted to direct her or criticize her driving, bite your tongue. Draw blood if necessary.

BACHELOR PARTIES

In recent years there's been so much nonsense written about the so-called inability of men to express their feelings to one another, and about macho chauvinist pigotry, that a sensible modern male might be tempted to forgo anything so atavistic, at least in stereotypical caricature, as the bachelor party. A sensitive guy is not supposed to enjoy an all-male gathering where the primary goals are to eat rare steaks, get knee-walking drunk, and ogle voluptuous strippers as they get down to bare essentials. So he begs off when his pals try to organize a bash on his behalf. That's a pity, since rites of passage—and what greater passage is there between birth and death than the step down the aisle from bachelor to husband?—sum up and underscore important stages of life. Getting together with your closest male friends, celebrating that special bond, recalling the moments together that make your friendship special, and affirming its future growth despite a sea change in one of your lives—why give up that just because the bachelor party has a tawdry connotation and unattractive history?

The trick is to replace the bachelor party stereotype with an event specially tailored to the ties that bind the groom and his friends together. If the erstwhile bachelor and his pals have been playing cards together every other Wednesday since college, a black-tie, all-night poker game at a swank downtown hotel with a professional dealer and champagne at the ready is the next best thing to flying to Las Vegas for the weekend, and a splendid way to salute the guest of honor. If you all share an obsession for pursuing the dimpled pellet, then hold the bachelor party at a resort hotel with a championship golf course. If the gang customarily congregates every weekend for two hours of hoops, then rent a giant screen (great) or fly to the site (greatest) and build the bachelor party around Final Four Saturday, even if it means shifting the wedding day or pretending you're single for the weekend. (Note: If you don't know what "Final Four Saturday" is, then pick another organizing principle.)

So long as you all remain in character, and stay true to the standards and values that brought you together in the first place, a bachelor party will reflect all your best qualities. Nowhere is it written that you can't have a good time with dear friends to celebrate your friendship.

Let the good times roll.

BAR MANNERS

The first thing to check out when entering a strange saloon is whether there is money lying on the bar. No money means the establishment runs a written tab to be paid upon departure. Bills and coins in front of patrons' glasses mean that you should toss down some cash after you order your drink but before the bartender returns with it. Chances are you'll feel more at home more quickly in a money-on-the-bar joint than in a tab place, so long as you don't expect to pay with a credit card. The bartender will collect what's due when he serves you, and will continue to do so as your thirst requires. Replenish the cash pile as needed, but don't touch it otherwise until you're ready to leave. Pocketing your change just to visit the men's room, for example, is tantamount to saying that your drinking companions right and left are thieves.

What's that? You say there's more to be said about bar manners? Probably. But only a couple of things come to mind, and you know them already: Never go to a bar expecting to drown your sorrows or to meet the woman of your dreams—it's a dead solid cinch you'll wind up disappointed.

Best Man

How do you tell who's the Best Man at the wedding? He's the only guy in a tux who's smiling. But enough wedding humor. What does the Best Man *really* do, aside from trying not to be better looking than the groom?

Well, in days gone by, when weddings were conducted by Robert's Rule of Nuptial Order, the Best Man had a number of clearly defined tasks: organizing the bachelor party (see BACHELOR PARTIES), driving the groom to the wedding, carrying the ring, keeping getaway plans secret, having a flask at the ready in case the groom is suddenly stricken by weak knees, and serving as legal witness to the ceremony.

Times have changed. Maybe it was the Sixties, with barefoot bride and groom exchanging vows of peace and garlands of flowers on a hilltop at sunset, and with the Grateful Dead replacing Mendelsohn, that caused the wedding rule book to be thrown away once and for all. Nowadays, maybe its the young upwardly mobile calculation that the poor risk-reward ratio of marriage makes pouring a whole lot of energy into an elaborate ceremony a poor investment. Who knows?

But while the precious role of the Best Man is no longer subject to clear definition, his overall responsibility is still crystal clear: to give general support to the groom-to-be. This could mean anything from lending a sympathetic ear to last-minute fears and doubts, to making sure that old friends aren't inadvertently left off the wedding list, to just being on call—a man for a man to talk to in time of need. Plus all the traditional tasks itemized above, of course.

One cautionary note: Picking a best man can be tricky business. A man with two or three particularly close friends is bound to disappoint someone, and if he has a couple of brothers, he could be causing filial pain to boot. A divorced man with children from an earlier marriage—and you run into a lot of both these days—can finesse the question by having his kids stand up with him as Best People. But there is often no obvious or easy way out of such a dilemma. Just remember that the earlier you deal with it by designating your best man (and, if the size of the wedding warrants it, assigning other duties to those passed over), the sooner any hurt feelings will fade away.

Question: If the groom's best friend (other than his bride, of course) happens to be a woman, is there any reason why she shouldn't stand up with him as his Best Person? None that we can think of, even if it is sure to generate a lot of whispering among aunts and uncles on both sides of the aisle.

Birth Control

Until the two of you jointly and explicitly decide otherwise, it's your responsibility.

BLACK TIE

Penguin jokes notwithstanding, a tuxedo—what mere mortals mean when they say black tie—is the Platonic ideal of clothing. When you put one on, you feel taller, broader of shoulder, narrower of hip, and tanner. Many are overcome by the impulse to say, "The name's Bond . . . James Bond." All women love men in tuxedos, and for that and lots of other good reasons we suggest you wear one every chance you get.

Used to be that you had to wait for a prom, a wedding, or some other occasion at which you wished you were dead, but that's all changed now. It's perfectly acceptable these days to don a tuxedo for the theater, the opera, the ballet, or even dinner at a nice restaurant. (Be sure to tell your companion for the evening what your plans are. There's no point in wearing tails if she is going to show up in cut-offs.) The worst thing that can happen is that the people around you will think you're on your way to or from an even swankier do.

Tuxedo rental is all right for the junior prom, but the sooner you stop wearing somebody else's clothes, the better. If you do rent, at least buy your own shirt—white, cotton, no ruffles, heavy on the starch. And start saving your pennies for the big time. Buying a tuxedo is probably the most enjoyable shopping experience you'll ever have. Give yourself a couple of hours in a slow season, go to the best clothing store you can afford, and make friends with the salesclerk and the tailor. You're going to have to make some hard choices (five minutes ago you didn't know there *were* different kinds of collars, and now you have to pick a favorite), but take comfort in the fact that you really can't go wrong if you chose what appeals to you and stay with black.

If you're not happy unless you're sporting a spot of color, go crazy with the tie and/or cummerbund. If you aspire to be thought eccentric or English, or both, be creative with the suspenders. Don't fool with the socks or shoes, though; stay with thin black dress socks and serious black shoes that tie. For the most festive of occasions Fred Astaire swears by patent leather. And we swear by Fred Astaire.

Real gold or onyx studs and cuff links would be perfect, but they may represent a greater commitment to formal wear than you are ready for. If so, any elegant but discreet jewelry that will keep you battened down will do nicely.

BLIND DATE

Why, when everyone in the world has at least one horror story about a blind date, do you keep giving them a try? Because you never know, that's why. And because there comes a time in every man's life when he has run out of co-workers and party invitations and he doesn't feel like dating the guy who delivers the pizza. And because for every twenty or so horror stories there's the greatest love story of our time, the one you tell your kids about on your wedding anniversary. So, once again, with fingers crossed and breath bated, you let yourself get fixed up.

When it happens again—and it will—keep in mind the following Things to Do and Not to Do on a Blind Date:

- Don't double date, even if your friend thinks it's a good idea. It's bad enough going through this without having spectators. Get her number from your friend, and make sure she's expecting your call. You take over from there.

- When you call, introduce yourself and tell her how you got her name and number. You've heard so much about her, you say, and all of it is of course so flattering that when you ask her out, she can't resist saying yes.

- Whatever you do, don't plan too long an evening. If you suggest dinner, the theater, and then dancing, you're in big trouble if you hate each other by the crème caramel.

- Don't choose anything too exotic. No matter how much you like cockfights or mud wrestling, it's just possible that she'll be put off.

- Don't forget the lunch date. The lighting probably isn't the greatest, but there are many places in which the atmosphere is fine. And perhaps most important, it takes just long enough for you to figure out if this is the real thing or if you want to murder your friend.

- At your first meeting, a little flattery never hurts. Be

on your best behavior even if someone has made a Terrible Mistake.

• Your obligations don't include having to see her again, but if you'd like to, give her a hint at the end of your first date. "May I see you again some time next week?" is as good a way as any. If she says yes, score one for the blind date; if she says no but has a good excuse, there may be hope; if she says she'd love to but she's planning to rearrange her sock drawer, someone's friend is in Big Trouble.

(See also DATING and LUNCH DATE.)

BREAD-AND-BUTTER GIFTS

A houseguest should always give his host and/or hostess a gift. There are no strict rules about when; it's fine to present something the minute you get there, any time during your stay, or soon (*very* soon) after you leave. (The truly practical houseguest chooses the first or second because it saves postage, but others find it easier to gather ideas for the perfect gift during their stay.)

We don't feel entirely comfortable telling you what to buy for your friends, but since our advice may mean that you'll be considered a gracious, well-mannered guest instead of a thoughtless ingrate, we'll take our chances. Keep in mind that the longer you stay and the more your hosts do for you, the nicer and more generous your gift should be. Here are six suggestions, in ascending order:

1. A bottle of good brandy.
2. A vase and a dozen roses.
3. Some fine caviar with all the trimmings.
4. A coffee grinder and some exotic coffee beans.
5. A great movie on videotape—you can't go wrong with *Citizen Kane* or *Gone with the Wind.*
6. A mixed case of wine.

If you object to buying bread-and-butter gifts, stay in a hotel. Better yet, stay home.

BREAKING DATES

If you're good at breaking dates, it can only mean you're doing it too often. It should be tough, something you do so rarely that you never master the knack.

We're talking here about breaking a social engagement, not canceling a business meeting you need more time to prepare for. And breaking it because you've changed your mind, not because you've been called away to Lisbon on a secret mission or given a ticket to the seventh game of the World Series. (Situations like that are so perfectly cut-and-dried that your erstwhile date will certainly understand. Or else.)

No, the tough case is when you have a date next Thursday with Ms. Maybe and—how to put it gracefully?—something better comes along.

What you do is up to you and your conscience, thank goodness. (Now don't you wish you'd read your Camus a little more thoughtfully?) *How* you do it concerns us here.

Honesty is the best policy, but only if you're prepared never to see the person you're stiffing again, and you're indifferent to her feelings. Let's look at the alternatives.

Lying is not the answer. You're going to feel a bit like a heel anyway—why feel like a liar, as well? No one goes through life without lying some, of course, but the more you look to it as a solution, the more it will come around to bite you in tender places.

It may help to reflect on how you've felt, and how you've behaved, when someone has broken a date with you. For one thing, it will tell you that no matter how creative your explanation or how smooth your delivery, the number of people in the world who'd like to punch you in the snoot is about to increase by one.

If you decide to break the date, then break it—but with no explanation of why, only a suggested alternative. "Look, I'm not going to be able to make it next Thursday after all. I'm sorry. Can we go out on Tuesday instead?" If she says yes, this is a good time for flowers (see FLOWERS). If she says no, then that's your tough luck.

The closer to the date, the greater risk you run of an explosion at the other end of the telephone—and rightly so. And it's one thing if the date is for the movies and a burger afterward, quite another if it's a dinner party at the Kissingers'.

Be prepared to answer the obvious question, "Why?" when you say that next Thursday's off. You'll be tempted, but resist the impulse to conjure up an urgent message from Woody Allen for a bedside visit with a sick script. Try to get by with, "Sorry, there's a personal matter I simply must attend to." If that flies, and Ms. Maybe turns out someday to be Ms. Right, you can both look back and have a laugh about it. Someday.

If you're in luck, of course, the "why" question won't come up, and you'll have gotten away—this one time—with having your cake and eating it.

BREAKING THE ICE

You enter a crowded room, arm yourself with something cold, and angle toward a neutral corner to rally your nerves. Suddenly you're intercepted by your hostess, who throws a hammerlock on your free arm. "There's someone I'm just dying for you to meet," she says. *I'm just dying,* you say to yourself. Seconds later you're face to face with a stranger, whose name you didn't quite hear and whose face has just clouded over with the look usually reserved for suspected airplane hijackers. Meanwhile, your hostess has hied off to mismatch two other poor souls, and you're left to your own devices. After you've repeated introductions to get the names straight (you don't want to go through your life as a "Gary" unless you are one), sorted out how each of you came to know your host and hostess, and agreed that it sure is warm in here, you discover that you've left your other devices at home.

Sound familiar? That's because breaking the ice is a social skill that ranks right up there with the ability to hum, accurately, a 10-year-old Stephen Sondheim song.

How you broke the ice used to depend on the sex of the other party. A man was a potential rival, a woman a potential breakfast companion, with conversational openers tailored accordingly. To a man, you usually talked about sports and job. With a woman, you might have solicited her opinion on the networks bidding for the new sitcom you were producing (anything to make you shine).

No more. A large social gathering is difficult enough to handle without turning it into a schoolyard turf fight or a fern-bar hustle. From now on, no separate conversational gambits for men and women. After all, your only goal should be to stimulate a few minutes of pleasant conversation. Power and sex can wait.

The best way to move things off dead center is with a non-threatening question. "What do you do?" is too blunt. The other person might hate his or her current job, or—worse still—might have just lost it. Politics and religion are off limits, at least until you determine whether the person has any. Specific questions ("Do you think Resnais has really grown since *Last Year at Marienbad?*") about movies, art, theater, and music are premature, and general queries ("Do you like movies?") make you sound like a simpleton stumped for anything to say.

The best ice-breaker, in an age where everybody is always moving around, is "Where are you from?" Geography is the most neutral of subjects, but is pregnant with conversational possibilities. Finding out that someone has moved here from Kansas three years ago, or grew up in Montana, or just got back from a year in Paris, opens up a whole range of secondary questions, allows you to compare impressions of places where paths have crossed, and prompts you both to explain how you came to be where you are.

More than that depends on chemistry.

BREAKING UP

They didn't write that song for nothing, you know. It *is* hard to do, particularly for the one who is on the receiving end of the bad news—and it's no trip to Hawaii for the bearer of the tidings either.

Let's face it, there's no good way to end a relationship, but some ways are better than others. (It's bad enough that you're calling it quits; you don't want to make it worse by behaving like a coward or a cad.) Although you probably won't come out of the situation with a huge fan club, if you follow these guidelines you'll minimize your risk of becoming the subject of cocktail party anecdotes or showing up as the villain in her first novel.

Be honest, but not painfully honest. This is not the time to recapitulate her shortcomings or tell her how to improve herself. Whenever possible, take the blame and take it like a man. Do it in person—no phone calls or notes, ever—but not necessarily in private. A public place is perfectly all right, but keep in mind that the confrontation may well be upsetting, so you won't want crowds. (A coffee house or a park will do as well as anyplace.) Don't try to cushion the blow with a lavish gift or an expensive meal or a sentimental trip down memory lane. You're probably already feeling guilty enough.

We hate to bring it up, but there may be times when you'll be on the receiving end of the bad news. With luck she'll have read the above beforehand, and with a little more luck you won't disgrace yourself, at least not publicly. The best advice we can give you about being dumped is: Do *not* write her a letter about how you feel, no matter how much you want to. That letter will haunt you to your dying day. (Okay, if you can't resist, go ahead and write the letter but *don't mail it.*) Otherwise we'll leave you alone to lick your wounds.

You may or may not reach the stage of being friends with your former girlfriend. Your social life will be less fraught with tension if you do, but even if you don't, you'll live. Avoid her if you can, and when you can't, don't talk about anything besides the weather or professional wrestling. Everything else will remind you of the time you spent together.

(See also LUNCH DATE.)

CHILDREN

Yes, they should probably be seen and not heard, but life is not like that, and neither are most kids. Whether they're yours or somebody else's, children can be a handful. A few basic rules should come in handy.

YOURS

One minute you're sitting in a coffee shop trying to keep them from throwing applesauce and making a scene that will get you thrown out of the joint. The next minute you're trying to restrain yourself from throttling their little-league coach. And the next thing you know you're screaming over the blare of their stereo about how bad loud music is for their hearing. Yup, as Roseanne Roseannadanna said, "It's always something."

We're not going to begin to try to give you the basics of child-rearing in these pages. Here we're concerned only with protocol, which can be boiled down to one strict rule: Do not assume that your children are welcome wherever you go. You love 'em, but let's face it—others, particularly childless others, may well think that they're a pain in the neck. Even if you're told that your children are welcome at an adult gathering, do everyone a big favor and leave them home.

Read our lips: GET A BABYSITTER.

If you're a divorced father, it's not always easy to introduce your kids to a new woman in your life. It probably makes sense not to go put your kids or yourself through it with casual dates; hold off until you've met someone who's going to be around for a while.

SOMEBODY ELSE'S

In general it's a lot easier to spend time with other people's kids than it is to hang out with your own. Tics and personality quirks that make you want to put your child up for adoption are usually funny or endearing or both in someone else's.

Still, if you're not used to kids, relating to them can make you feel old and awkward. For the novice, a few Dos and Don'ts:

- DON'T ask how school is. Kids hate that.
- DON'T tell a kid how tall he's getting. They hate that too.
- DON'T try too hard to be a real pal. They'll think you're a jerk.
- DON'T make it your business to draw a child out. Pay attention, sure, but don't press it.
- DON'T lecture or hold forth on how things were when you were his age. They're not interested in you unless you're a rock star or a regular on *Miami Vice,* or unless you can fix it so that they can buy leather jackets, motorcycles, and U-2 tapes at wholesale prices.
- All the above notwithstanding, *DO* make an effort to have some contact with kids—a girlfriend's nephews, the neighbor's quintuplets, whatever. We're not saying you have to rush right out and coach little league, but we are saying that it's healthy to spend at least a little of your time with people who aren't your age. Besides, having kids around gives you an excuse for going to the circus or seeing again *101 Dalmatians.*

CHRISTMAS CARDS

Hallmark will deny it to the death, but the fact is that the Christmas card may well be going the way of the appendix and the goony bird. Nowadays everybody is sending and receiving fewer Christmas cards and enjoying them less. Even businesses that have traditionally sent out hundreds year after year are starting to wonder whether the time and money involved might be better spent on a new water cooler.

While this turn of events may cause some of us to sigh and make joyful noises about caroling, eggnog, ribbon candy, and other swell things about Christmas past, it's easy to understand how all this happened. First of all, the telephone has made virtually all personal correspondence pretty rare (see LETTERS). Second, people don't often send cards to people they often see or to whom they're giving a gift. (See GIFTS.) And third, empty sentiment took quite a beating in the Sixties, and it's never quite recovered. (Nine out of ten baby boomers think that mass mailings of printed Christmas cards are dopey.)

What's more, it's sort of hard to mourn the passing of the kinds of Christmas cards that used to fill our mailboxes—the imprinted card, the form letter, and the one with the picture of Mom, Dad, the kids, and the pet hamster.

All this Scrooge-like carping notwithstanding, sending your heartfelt holiday greetings is a thoughtful gesture, and your loved ones will certainly appreciate it very much. Just be sure that you enclose a personalized note with each card you decide to send. If it's not worth taking the time to say a few sincere words, it's really not worth sending.

CLEANING HELP

They used to be called maids or cleaning women or just "help," but now who knows what you're supposed to call them? By whatever name, the important thing is to call them, since housemaid's knee is now what most of us have in mind when we think about the scars of battle. It follows that you have to know how to behave when a cleaning person shows up.

But first, the search for the perfect cleaning help. To find someone who will baby your golf trophies and at the same time make sure that penicillin is not rediscovered in your shower, ask around. Agencies are fine, but if you're going to allow strangers to separate your socks, there is no substitute for the recommendation of a friend.

The day she (let's assume it's a she) arrives for the first time, show her around, tell her what you would like her to do, give her quarters for the washer and dryer, and then leave her to it. Some men feel better if a female friend is there the first day, and while we don't condone this kind of backsliding, we do understand and accept it. (You're not allowed to have your mother there, though. We have some standards.)

If you do decide to handle negotiations yourself, bear in mind that sometimes it's not just windows they don't do. Some don't do laundry, iron, or polish silver, either. Even if you don't care too much about the specifics, you should at least work them out in advance, perhaps offering a little more cash ($5 to $8 per hour is the range, but ask around to find out what your friends are paying) for extra chores. You're responsible for cleaning equipment, but she's in charge of making sure you know what she needs. Leave something to eat and drink in the refrigerator. If your schedule is flexible, you can probably let her in each week, but if not, ask a neighbor to do so or, better yet, give her a key.

Don't expect to be able to use your kitchen as an O.R. when

you get home, but you ought to be able to tell that someone with some ammonia and a mop has been there. And don't squawk if your root beer is gone.

(See also HOUSEWORK.)

COCKTAIL PARTIES

Anything that's hot, noisy, and smoky and demands that we hold a drink and a stuffed mushroom and shake somebody's hand at the same time will never make it to our list of favorite activities. And those are just some of the problems with cocktail parties. Another: You never know enough people there, and those you do know are boring and trap you in conversation for what seems like hours. In short, most cocktail parties are about as appealing as root canal, and we can't imagine why anyone would willingly attend one.

But attend you (and, alas, we) will. What's more, one day you may find yourself hosting one.

Herewith a few words about both.

WHEN YOU'RE THE GUEST

It's always possible that this cocktail party will be one of the few great ones, but just in case it isn't, it can help if you keep a few protective measures in mind:

• Arrive about a half hour after you're asked and leave a half hour before the end. If the invitation says 6:00 to 8:00, stay from 6:30 to 7:30. If you're invited for 6:00 but not told when to go home, stay no longer than an hour and a half. For more about this, see TAKING YOUR LEAVE.

• Say hello and goodbye to your host, but don't expect him/her to spend a lot of time with you. Cocktail parties do not provide quality time—with anyone. The idea here is to make some sort of contact with as many people as possible in a short period of time while not spilling anything. If it's meaningful interaction with strangers you want, try group therapy.

• Don't try to make a meal out of the refreshments. Serious nibbling is perfectly okay, but it's unseemly to be caught stuffing your pockets with fistfuls of cashews or pigs-in-a-blanket.

• Mix. You're not the host, but as a good guest you have a responsibility to hold up your end. Talk to everyone you already know and then force yourself to talk to at least one stranger. If you want to be eligible for the Good Samaratin award, pick someone who seems particularly ill at ease and make pleasant conversation for at least five minutes.

- Unless this is a business party, don't identify yourself by describing what your job is. Talk about your host (asking how the stranger comes to know him/her is good for a minute or two) or other neutral but not unduly deadening topics. (For suggestions about conversation with strangers, see BREAKING THE ICE.)

WHEN YOU'RE THE HOST

No matter how much you don't exactly love cocktail parties, the time may come when you want to bring together a large number of people without feeding them a meal. It is then that only a cocktail party will do. Here's how to make yours better than most:

- Invite—with written invitations—about half again as many people as you have room for and try to get a pretty good idea of how many people will eventually show. (See RSVP for advice on how to get answers out of people.) In general, the more crowded a cocktail party is, the better it is; people have to mix if they're leaning against one another. Don't be too picky about numbers, though. There will be plenty of unexpected no-shows, but there will also undoubtedly be some unexpected friends of friends. Have plenty of food and drink and go with the flow.

- Keep the room cool. Lots of bodies and lots of smoke make for a hot, stuffy room in a hurry. Be prepared with fans, air conditioners, open windows, whatever.

- Never *ever* throw a cocktail party and then serve only one kind of beverage, especially if you're thinking of making it white wine. It's okay to have a specialty of the house (especially if it's a mean margarita), but be sure that anything within reason is also available. Make friends with your liquor store and get some advice on what constitutes a fully stocked bar (see LIQUOR CABINET). Don't worry about buying too much—most stores will be happy to take back unopened bottles.

- Hire help, as much as you can afford. The minimum: a bartender and someone who will carry around trays of food during the party and clean up afterwards.
- Serve food but don't try to get written up by *Gourmet* magazine. It should taste good, hold up well on a tray for a couple of hours, be substantial enough to keep the heavy drinkers from keeling over, and not be too messy when balanced with a drink. Consider nachos, little meatballs, or—if money is no object—shrimp.
- Think about the music in advance—nothing too loud, nothing too sleepy or funereal. Records are bound to get scratched, so tapes are your best bet.
- The party's over, it's time to call it a day, and you're stuck with a few stragglers. There's a Nobel Prize in it for you if you can figure out the perfect way to get rid of them. A few imperfect ways are saying good night and then leaving yourself (not too friendly), inviting everyone out to dinner (expensive), closing the bar (which may make you look like a piker), and turning off the lights (which might make you look rude). Probably the best thing is to wait them out as graciously as possible. After all, maybe this means you had a good party!

COHABITATION

L iving together is not the same as being married, no matter what anyone says. It's close, though—just short of saying it's for keeps—and the success of the arrangement is just as dependent on proper behavior as marriage is. If you're thinking about taking the medium-sized plunge, there are several things to remember.

You may not be married, but you do have an understanding. The days of complete freedom are over, and while you don't have to spend all of your time together, it's only polite that you keep each other informed about where you are and what you're doing. (If you are going out with friends, she doesn't absolutely have to be invited, but she does have to be told about it.) And needless to say, you are no longer dating.

Your house is her house, and that means that you both cook in it, clean it, decorate it, and entertain in it. That also means that you let each other know in advance if visitors are expected. There are all sorts of ways to divide cooking and cleaning chores, so you'll have to find one that suits you both. (See HOUSE-WORK for more about the division of labor.)

Joint checking accounts and such come with orange blossoms and a gold band (if they come at all), but joint ownership usually begins with living together. If your incomes are identical, you will probably want to go fifty-fifty on expenses, but if not, get out your calculator and come up with a system that works. Even if you outearn her, you're not her personal banker or loan officer. (And she's not yours, even if she's a stockbroker and you're a street musician.) Remember, the two major causes of arguments in any relationship are money and sex.

Be sure to keep track of who owns what. We're as romantic as the next guy, but we can't ignore the possibility that one of these days your house will not be her house and the property will have to be divided. This doesn't mean labeling your place mats and measuring spoons; it does mean having an understanding about who owns the tape deck and the coffee table.

COMPLIMENTS

It's a real puzzlement how something that should be terrific to give and (especially) to get can cause so much discomfort to absolutely everyone concerned. But it's true: Most people find it hard to give and to receive even the simplest compliment.

GIVING THEM

If you can remember how uncomfortable you sometimes feel when you're on the receiving end of a compliment, it can make you a lot better at doling them out. The basic rule here is to be generous and sincere without being excessive. Don't overpraise or give undeserved compliments, but when you do see something you like, say so, as in: "I thought you did a wonderful job on that presentation," or "That's a great-looking dress," or "Your apartment is beautiful," or "This is the best pecan pie I've ever tasted." And *don't* give compliments to get something—a promotion, a roll in the hay, a mention in the will—in return. It doesn't usually work, and it will make you feel like a sycophant. And so it should.

GETTING THEM

Respond to any and all compliments with two simple words: "Thank you." No muss, no fuss, no "Oh, this crummy old rag?" or "It was nothing, really" or "Anyone could have done it" or "I got it on sale" or "It could have been a lot better if . . ." or "Do you really think so?" Just "Thank you." If that doesn't seem like enough, you can say "Thank you very much." Then change the subject.

COOKING

The hoary caricature of the bachelor who can't boil water and never enters his kitchen except to get another beer still crops up in black-and-white TV reruns, but it has no place in modern life. A man should be at least as adept at preparing food as he is at selecting his own wardrobe. Helplessness is not cool.

If you can read, you can cook, so there's no reason for not being able to handle kitchen basics. This does not mean spending all your disposable income on kitchen equipment or taking a tutorial from Julia Child. It does mean knowing how to prepare an intimate supper for two *and* a formal (okay, *semi*formal) dinner for eight. (See also HOST, DINNER PARTY, SETTING A TABLE, WINE, and LIQUOR CABINET.)

For starters, use cloth napkins at every meal unless the main course is barbecued spareribs. Permanent press—the miracle process you want to keep away from your shirts—makes this feasible. Even picnics taste better if you have a cloth napkin on your lap. Look better, too.

You can get by nicely with half a dozen good recipes. (Where you get them is up to you, but James Beard and Craig Claiborne are good places to start.) You should, for example, learn how to make a perfect vinaigrette dressing (that plus fresh greens, a great loaf of bread, and a chunk of good cheese make a perfect summer meal), know how long to cook pasta (not very), how to turn out a perfect omelet to accompany the champagne in a late supper, and how to roast leg of lamb to feed six to eight at dinner. (Roast 15 to 18 minutes per pound at 350 degrees; let sit for a half hour outside the oven before carving. Yes, it's that easy.)

Steam vegetables 8 to 10 minutes. Bake potatoes 50 minutes at 400 degrees. Broil fish 10 minutes per inch in thickness. Add one cup rice to two cups boiling water, add one teaspoon salt, cover and simmer for 20 minutes. Serve cheese and fruit at room temperature.

Simple? Exactly. And the simpler your cooking is (at least at first), the better. There's no need to make a fetish out of eating, but there's also no reason to believe it can be done only at a restaurant or someone else's home. *Bon appetit!*

CREDIT CARDS

These days you'd be crazy not to want to master the possibilities, positively nuts to think about leaving home without it. We're with Benjamin's adviser in *The Graduate* all the way—plastic is aces.

However, credit cards are not merit badges, and whether they're gold, platinum, or Black Watch plaid, they're not meant to be flaunted. By all means use them, but don't brandish them. To save embarrassment (not to mention dishpan hands) call ahead to make sure that the restaurant of your choice accepts the credit card of your choice.

If you've gone out to dinner, and you're planning to split a fairly hefty tab, you don't need to argue over who'll pay cash and who'll get to use his or her credit card. Many restaurants will quite happily take two cards and put half the bill on each. Isn't progress wonderful?

(See also MONEY)

DANCING

We don't like to be pessimistic, but we have to say it: If you haven't learned how to dance yet, you probably never will. You might give dancing lessons a try, but don't be surprised if they turn out to be a waste of money. It's sad but true—some men have it and some men don't. Alas, most women do.

If you don't, the occasions at which it is necessary to demonstrate your shortcomings are mercifully few and far between. Thank your lucky stars you're not traveling on your two left feet through Tara and Twelve Oaks with Miz Scarlett. (Even Ashley Wilkes could dance, and no one was a bigger wimp than Ashley.) And while you're being grateful, keep in mind that modern dances are a lot easier to master than the dances of yore. It's tough to fake a minuet, but if pressed, most men can learn a halfway decent box step and fox trot, too. You'll save yourself a lot of embarrassment if you spend a few hours at it.

So there's no reason to be proud that when it comes to tripping the light fantastic, you're mostly tripping, but you don't have to hang your head in shame either. Avoid dancing whenever you can, but don't shirk your responsibilities when you can't.

Those responsibilities include dancing with your hostess, your date (who should know in advance that you don't dance and be free to dance with others), and all the women at your table at least once. No one can expect more than that.

DATING

Until the day comes when some genius (destined to enjoy great wealth and the unlimited admiration of his peers) dreams up a new method by which members of the opposite sex can get acquainted, we're all stuck with a system that is, at best, imperfect: dating.

The feminist movement promised to make things a lot better, more relaxed, and take some of the heat off men (Great! Women calling men for dates! And picking up the check!), but whatever changes did occur were merely temporary. Dating is still—dating.

The protocol of dating hasn't changed much since your dad drove you to pick up cute little What's-Her-Name to take her to the Bijou and the Dairy Queen. Unless you have a good reason to behave otherwise, you still do the inviting (and risk the rejection), and you still pay the bills.

The good news is that when you pay and you do the asking, you get to choose where you want to go. But use your power wisely—you're more likely to have company on a regular basis if you line up activities that she's likely to enjoy too.

It's no longer considered necessary to pick her up at her place at the beginning of the date, but you still should be prepared to see her safely home afterward. If you never want to see her again, don't call, but if you do, be sure to give her a buzz the next day, to tell her so.

And you're *still* not supposed to kiss and tell.

(See also DINNER DATE, LUNCH DATE, FIRST DATE, BLIND DATE, and BREAKING DATES.)

DINNER DATE

The primary purpose of a dinner date—at least in the first stages of a relationship—has little to do with food, even less with ancillary entertainment, and everything with getting to know each other. With that principle firmly in mind, you'll have a good head start on what *not* to do.

Don't go to a theme restaurant. You know, where all the waiters dress up like pirates or Renaissance balladeers or something, and the menus are written entirely in cute.

Don't ask your date, "What kind of food do you like?" Food is not the point, remember, and what if she likes nothing better than a whopping great porterhouse, medium rare, and you haven't eaten red meat since 1981? If the dinner date was your idea, you pick the place. Do tell her in advance where you are going, since she needs time to decide how to dress, and an opportunity to sound the alarm if you've picked the place where she and her former love staged a loud and tearful breakup.

Don't select a trendy hot spot. The last thing you want to do is stand at a packed bar until 9:15 when you have dinner reservations at 8:00. The trendier the place, the longer the wait (and, increasingly, the worse the service—and the food). Anyway, since when did you want to be leader of the pack?

Don't leave the mainstream. If things work out, you'll have plenty of time to explore your individual preferences in exotic cuisine together. If the special appetizer is roast sheepshead, she may be out the door before your waiter gets to the main course.

Don't go to a dinner theater. Ever.

Don't pick a restaurant with a piano player. Or strolling violinists, or singing waiters, or—God help you!—an accordionist. Music has its place, and sometimes that's even in a restaurant. But not when you're trying to find out what she thinks about baseball.

Don't go to the fanciest, most expensive four-star gourmet restaurant in town. Save that for your first anniversary together. Why blow a fortune on what may, after all, be your last date?

The best place for a dinner date? That's easy. It's a restaurant where you've been before, where you like the atmosphere and food, and where you're comfortable. Note the emphasis on "you." That's because your being as much at ease as possible is the best hope for the date to be more than just dinner.

DINNER PARTY

Forget graduation and your first kiss. The rite of passage that puts them all to shame is your first dinner party. Heaven knows you've been to enough of them, for business and for pleasure, in large groups and small, but it's just not the same as throwing one yourself.

In many ways it's a lot better to be the host than to be the guest. You get to pick the guest list, decide on the seating plan, and choose the wine. You don't have to eat lima beans or aspic. You can have cocktails for as long as you like, and your favorite brand of coffee. On the other hand, you have to put fresh towels in the bathroom and set the table, and you don't get to turn in until everyone goes home. And then there's the matter of dishes.

No question about it—throwing dinner parties can be a lot like hard work. But it also brings satisfactions that you just can't get from picking up the tab at a restaurant.

The trick is to keep the whole thing simple. Unless you're actually opening a small restaurant, never have more than eight people around the table. Six is really the optimum number, especially for novices. Plan on serving dinner at 8:30 and invite people for 7:30. (Learn to make a mean martini or a perfect margarita and maybe a dip for chips and vegetables. That kind of thing takes no time at all but can make all the difference.)

Before your guests arrive, be sure that the place is clean (see HOUSEWORK and CLEANING HELP) and the table is set (forks and napkins on the left, knives and wineglasses on the right, flowers and/or candles in the center), and that the wine and salad greens are chilled. No one minds if you bang a few pots around, but it's a trifle unseemly to scour the bathtub once your audience has arrived. Choose the music you want to hear, if any. Nowhere is it written that you must have background music, but many people feel that strains of Schubert or Willie Nelson can fill an awkward silence. (On the other hand, heavy metal is for your little brother, and Philip Glass is an acquired taste. Be careful.)

Gather all the serving dishes and utensils you'll eventually need. Take the butter out of the refrigerator. Grind the coffee.

You should also have a seating plan. You don't absolutely have to follow the boy-girl-boy-girl pattern, but it almost always makes sense, and couples shouldn't sit next to or directly across from each other. If there are singles at your table, you need not play matchmaker, but it may make sense to seat them next to each other. It will often be a good idea for you to have a female companion for the evening, if only for symmetry's sake. If you're between mature commitments at the moment, invite a friend to do the honors.

When people start showing up, either sit down with them and have a drink or suggest they join you in the kitchen if you're not ready to sit yet. Your chief responsibility during the cocktail hour is to introduce your guests and give them something to talk about while you're putting the finishing touches on the meal ("You know, Joe, Bill is almost as much of a fanatic about golf as you are. He's thinking about going to Pinehurst over Christmas. Weren't you there last year?"). Later, when you're seated around the table, you can let the conversation run a bit more freely, but it will remain your job to keep the conversational ball rolling. (If this proves to be impossibly hard, spend more time over the guest list next time. You need a nice mix of talkers and listeners.)

Now for the meal. Remember, simplicity is your byword. There's nothing wrong with serving elaborate dishes that take days to prepare, but do that sort of thing only if it gives you pleasure. The guests may appreciate a well turned-out terrine or classic puff pastry, but unless they've trained at the Cordon Bleu, they won't really know all the work that went into it. No, you're better off with something simple. Get yourself a few basic cookbooks and work on developing a specialty that's delicious and filling and can be made in advance. Beef stew comes first to mind, especially since in a pinch you can call it Boeuf Bourgignon. Coq au Vin—chicken in wine sauce—is another, and for the seafood lover in you there's Shrimp Creole. Any one-dish meal will suit your purposes nicely.

Add rice, a salad (learn how to make a decent vinaigrette—eight tablespoons oil, two tablespoons vinegar, a teaspoon of Dijon mustard, a half teaspoon of salt, and a couple of chopped garlic cloves), good bread, dessert (a terrific store-bought cheesecake is never wrong), and about half a bottle of wine per person, and you've got yourself the perfect dinner.

Now comes the moment of truth: Coffee is served. Freshly ground beans and freshly dripped coffee are best, but the critical element here is speed. The wine is gone, dessert is on the table, brandy awaits. The guests want coffee, and they want it NOW. If you're serving drip coffee, have the coffee measured into the container and the water measured out into the kettle before you sit down to eat. You might opt for investing in a coffee percolator, a virtually forgotten contraption in these days of home espresso machines. You might lose a few points for flavor, but you'll win plenty for timing.

As baby boomers jog toward Medicaid, more and more dinner guests are taking a pass on the coffee—can't stand the caffeine, too much acid, whatever. It's nice to have decaffeinated coffee, regular tea, and herb tea around for these occasions, and it's especially nice if you serve an alternative beverage without making a big deal of it.

With dinner parties, as with all things, practice makes perfect. The more dinners you have, especially if you serve the same few dishes all the time, the better you'll get at it. You'll also stop worrying about timing and start having fun.

Now all you need is brandy, cigars, and a drawing room.

(See also COOKING, WINE, LIQUOR CABINET.)

DIVORCE

No matter how much a divorce—yours or someone else's—complicates your life and makes you wish you'd never been born, just remember that it could be worse: You could be Edward VIII. You may have to say goodbye to a few friends, some furniture, and a part of your income, but with luck you won't have to give up the throne for the woman you love.

We couldn't hope to cover all of the emotional, financial, logistical, and spiritual ramifications of divorce here. What we can do is discuss the protocol of the most common situations that may crop up in the aftermath of a divorce.

YOUR FORMER WIFE

No one says you have to like her, although it's quite the thing these days to remain on friendly terms with your ex-wife. In fact, if your encounters are strictly private, for our purposes it doesn't much matter how you and she treat each other (despite the fact that it's childish, it can still be cathartic to rekindle old animosities every once in a while). But if your paths are wont to cross in public, you would do well to work out a way of relating to her that doesn't involve raised voices and high blood pressure. Divorce is many things, but it's not a spectator sport.

Even if it's completely phony, having a brief, bland prepared statement ("Hello. How are you? How are your folks/the kids? Good.") at the ready can save you from embarrassment and/or committing a gaffe when you and your former spouse accidentally run into each other. If she tries to discuss something a trifle less neutral, feel free to say, "I'd rather not talk about that here. Why don't you give me a call?" and leave it at that.

When you do run into an openly hostile former wife, if you're with someone—a friend, a date, male or female—it's not necessary to make introductions. If a divorce was unpleasant, sometimes even that is asking for trouble. However, most former wives may be treated as you would treat a distant relative. Warmth isn't required, but a certain cordiality is called for.

HER FORMER HUSBAND

Being involved with a divorced woman can also have its problems (see Edward VIII, above), but most of them can be solved by staying as far out of the way as you can if and when weapons are being chosen. Of course, if everyone has remained friends, there's probably nothing to worry about, but if not, keep in mind that it's not your place to intervene. Of course, you're on her side, but the idea is to make the choosing of sides unnecessary.

When you find yourself playing a bit part (or bigger) in a scene between a divorced couple, be as unobtrusive as possible. If you try to lighten the mood by cracking jokes or serving as go-between or goodwill ambassador, they'll both hate you. And who could blame them?

YOUR FRIENDS

Of all the casualties of a divorce, the ones who get relatively little press are the friends of the erstwhile happy couple. If life were perfect, everyone would be able to maintain all the pre-divorce friendships, but life (as you may have noticed) isn't. As a matter of fact, where divorce is concerned, there are times when it isn't even pleasant.

Once in a while you will be able to see both halves of a divorced couple, but more often you'll have to choose sides—or have them chosen for you. The most important thing to remember is that regardless of which half of the couple gets custody of you, you mustn't say anything rotten about the other half. You can listen, sure. You can even nod your head and look sympathetic. But you're treading on dangerous territory if you start reciting your own litany of complaints. Keep in mind that if they get married again, you want to be invited to the wedding.

Doors, Elevators, Escalators, Revolving Doors

These modern conveniences are supposed to make life easier, but of course they've also muddied the waters a bit. After all, a person wants to be polite, but a person still has to get to work on time. The problems usually start when in our efforts to be well-mannered we tend to forget our objectives. As it is in most things, in dealing with doors of all kinds, common sense is your strongest ally. For instance, if your arms are full of packages, there's no need to open a door with your nose.

Thanks to the feminist movement, there have been some changes in acceptable behavior when it comes to door-holding. With the exception of the handicapped, the elderly, and the pregnant—who always get preferred treatment—the holding of doors is now an equal opportunity activity.

DOORS

When you are walking with someone, male or female, whoever gets to a door first holds it open for the other. Don't race to be first, but don't be shy either. If the door opens in, life is simple: Pull the door toward you and wait until your companion walks through. If it opens out, you have a choice: Either push it out and wait, or push it out, walk through it, hold it, and wait.

ELEVATORS

When getting on, let others go first and then head to the back of the car. When getting off, let anyone in front of you go first, but don't worry about the folks behind you.

ESCALATORS

Ideally you let your companion go first when getting on an escalator, but then you get off first. (Nothing to it unless it's very crowded or you're paralyzed with fear. You simply move alongside of her in transit and then take the lead.) That way you can turn around to make sure that she gets off the escalator without any difficulty.

REVOLVING DOORS

Common sense says that you hop in the revolving door first so that you can get the door moving (or slow it down if necessary) for your companion, but he or she may be less sensible than you and may think that you're being rude. To be on the safe side, let her go first but give her a helpful little push to start. Just make sure you push *counter*clockwise.

DUTCH TREAT

Splitting the check is one of those amazing phenomena that manages to make everyone feel rotten. Penny-pinchers are sure they've paid for someone else's extra cup of coffee, glad-handers feel like penny-pinchers, and somebody always gets stiffed. Even the waiter looks miserable. If you're part of a large group and there's no way around it, at least don't start figuring who had the side order of onion rings; divide the check plus tip by the number of people paying and get the hell out of there.

If you're half of a couple, there's really no excuse for splitting the check. When in doubt, the man still pays. If she's got class (and a full-time job), she'll pick it up the next time or maybe the time after that. And because you're a with-it kind of guy, you'll let her.

ENGAGEMENT RING

It's just like in the movies. You kneel in front of her before the fireplace in her parents' living room, you ask her to close her eyes, you take her hand in yours, and you slip a ring onto the third finger of her left hand . . . only . . . only, no matter how you twist and shout, the damned thing won't go on!

This will come as a decidedly minor view, but we think that the pomp and circumstance surrounding getting married have gotten out of hand (see WEDDING). Unless you both come from royal families and have national obligations to discharge, why not celebrate and affirm your personal commitment to each other in a simple, quiet, *personal* way?

A good place to start is with the engagement. So far as we can tell, the formal announcement of a couple's intentions to marry was merely the excuse (once upon a time) to get down to brass tacks on the subject of dowry. The basic outlines had been agreed to previously, of course, but the interval between engagement and wedding was needed to dot the *i*'s and cross the *t*'s on the contract. Twenty cows or twenty-five? Three young mares or four? Stuff like that. Time was also needed for the bride's mother to sew the wedding dress and prepare her trousseau, but the main reason for a period of engagement was the redistribution of property and the restructuring of family alliances. Romance? Forget about it.

Now, we're not saying you shouldn't announce to friends and family your intention to get married. But consider this: It's hard to keep matters under control if the engagement—which is only Step One, after all—is a Big Bang Extravaganza. By the time you actually head up the middle aisle, you're both likely to be worn out (mentally and physically) from the premarital ordeal of it all.

Having said all that, we might as well go one step more and suggest that you consider taking a pass on the ring. Diamonds are forever, it's true, but marriages aren't, at least not in our times. Why sink the equivalent of a down payment on a good car on a bauble that only one of you, after all, gets to wear? Why not spend those bucks on, say, a down payment on a good car? Really, you give her a whopping great ring, she gives you a kiss. Is that fair? Is that sensible?

And what if it doesn't fit?

EXERCISE

Whether you stay in shape and, if so, how you do it are not our concerns here. The Surgeon General and Jane Fonda think it's a good idea, and we learned a long time ago that it's not smart to argue with them. No, we're interested here in the *etiquette* of fitness, which is the simplest aspect of it anyway.

Feel free to carry your squash racquet in crowded office elevators and wear shirts that show off your hard-won muscles and flat stomach, but never talk about the exercise you take unless you're specifically asked. And then as soon as you can manage it, change the subject.

No one really wants to hear how far or fast you run, how much iron you can pump, or how many laps you can swim, and it's almost unseemly to talk about such things in polite society. Your resting heart rate is no one's business but your own. So jump rope but keep quiet about it.

Health club etiquette depends on the club you choose. Some frown on socializing, while others are singles' bars with Nautilus machines and sweat bands. When in Rome . . .

FATHER'S DAY

Most men don't care much about Father's Day, or at least they pretend not to. (One father of seven we know has renamed it Old Spice Day and threatens to leave town once a year unless everyone gives him dark gray socks.) But of course they do care, and so should you—enough to send at least a card and preferably a gift as well. If you feel strongly that a telephone call is plenty, at least call early. If you don't, it could be a long, suspenseful day for Dad.

In gifts, money doesn't matter but thought goes a long way. If your dad is like a lot of others, he might enjoy a dozen golf balls, a good bottle of port, a tennis sweater, six kinds of ice cream toppings, or a good book. Not to mention dark gray socks.

FIRST DATE

S ome guys say that even blind dates are better than first dates, because with a blind date you can always look elsewhere for a scapegoat if it doesn't work out. In the case of a first date you're going out with someone who isn't a complete stranger. You've seen each other and at least had a conversation. If it's a disaster, you've nobody to blame but yourself.

However, there are some similarities between a first and a blind date, the most important of which is that in both you've got to get through that agonizing getting-to-know-each-other period. Time, place, and ambience are critical.

Forget the Super Bowl or a porn movie. Cultural events are all right, but Mozart and Neil Simon can get in the way of conversation. Dinner on a weeknight is good, but a weekday lunch may be even better. You don't have to pick her up at her place, but if it's conveniently located, you should offer to do so. (Some women wouldn't hear of it. Among other things they don't want a relative stranger in their apartments.)

If the date was your idea, you get to pick the restaurant, but it's only good manners to ask for her preference. Ideally you'll give her a choice, and when she says (as she should), "Either one sounds fine," suit yourself. That means someplace comfortable and quiet, neither the cheapest beanery nor the biggest prix fixe in town. Nice lighting, friendly waiters, and a good house wine can definitely ease the pain of a first date.

SIX THINGS NOT TO TALK ABOUT ON A FIRST DATE
1. Your old girlfriends
2. Sex
3. Disease
4. Professional wrestling
5. Your work (at least not much)
6. Money

SIX THINGS TO TALK ABOUT ON A FIRST DATE

1. Her
2. Your hometown
3. Food
4. Travel
5. Movies
6. Politics. It used to be taboo, but no more. Anyhow, if you're passionately opposed, better find out sooner than later.

EPILOGUE

There is no such thing as an automatic "I'll call you" after a first date. You don't have to—seeing her home and shaking her hand goodnight are all that's expected of you—but don't say you will if you won't. If you want to see her again but can't decide whether or not she'd like to hear from you, take a deep breath and ask her. A simple "May I call you later in the week?" will do the trick.

(See also BLIND DATE, LUNCH DATE, DATING, and BREAKING THE ICE.)

FLOWERS

A rose is a rose is a rose, and that's the problem. When most of us think of sending flowers, it's only to a lady fair, and then we reach for a dozen long stems the way Pavlov's dog responded to that bell. This has got to stop. Giving flowers is too wonderful a gesture to be governed by reflex action or to be restricted to the service of romance. Here are some guidelines for making the best of a good thing.

Deep background. For starters, you need to know what flowers mean. "There is an isomorphism between a flower and female genitalia," explains a prominent Manhattan psychoanalyst. "When a man gives a woman flowers, he's saying to her that her labia are as beautiful to him as the petals of a rose. He chooses a bud instead of a fully opened flower not just because it will last longer and give better value but because it suggests modesty and innocence. A single flower is more explicitly romantic because it is phallic, which is of course why a longer stem is preferred."

Of course. And you thought you were only buying a bunch of posies?

The source. The only way to feel confident in selecting flowers is to spend some time at a florist's shop. Not a farm-and-garden store that peddles fertilizer, shrubs, and peat moss along with a few flowers, but a place where the ratio of cut flowers to potted plants is at least 40 to 60. Eyeball everything, then ask the names of the ones you fancy—and take notes. Find out if your favorites are seasonal or if they're available year-round. Check out the kinds of cards that are attached to flowers ordered by telephone; you don't want an excellent choice tainted by a silly card bordered with cupids.

Nature's bounty. The reason for visiting a florist's shop is to see and smell first-hand the enormous variety of beautiful options to roses. If you think a peony is some sort of little horse, then freesias, Peruvian lilies, anemones, delphiniums, lilacs, and daffodils will be so many meaningless words if you don't see them for yourself at least once.

Arrangements. Steer clear of floral arrangements unless the occasion for the flowers is a funeral. Even then you're likely to be better off choosing a bunch of one flower than a hodgepodge of many stuck into a styrofoam base and padded with ferns. Any gift you give is an expression of yourself, so be wary of ceding the right of selection to a merchant whose primary goal is to move stock with a short shelf-life.

Occasions. The sobering truth is that most flowers sold in America end up in hospital rooms and funeral parlors. Surely a people that has walked on the moon can think of upbeat uses as well for something so certain to evoke smiles? The summer solstice, a moment of inspiration by your tax accountant, Bach's birthday, a promotion, a Cubs' pennant, and the fact that it's Tuesday are perfectly fine occasions for flowers. The best occasion of all? Whenever they're least expected. Don't wait for anniversaries or arguments.

Friendship. Nowhere is it written that you may not give flowers to a female friend without implying romance—or to a male friend, for that matter. The one constant about flowers is their ability to lift the human spirit. Why restrict arbitrarily the number of your friends to whom you can give such a boost?

Potted plants. For aunts and couples, never for lovers or spouses, and okay for friends *only* if you are one-hundred-percent sure they enjoy spending the time and attention some plants require. Keeping an African violet is tough work, and you don't want to end up being cursed every time a leaf dies.

Exceptions to that rule. Certain flowering plants—amaryllis, azaleas, and paper-white narcissus are examples—come in pots but make swell gifts because they don't just sit there and look green. As a courtesy to their recipient, be sure to check with your florist about proper care and feeding.

Corsages. Once *de rigueur* for many occasions, the corsage is now pretty well restricted to old-fashioned moms on Mother's

Day. Gone are the days when a young man would arrive at his sweetheart's doorstep with a boxed orchid under his arm.

Carnations. Forget the flower whose primary virtue is its virtual indestructibility. Red or white carnations are appropriate only in the lapels of high school boys on prom night and of grown men who want to draw attention to themselves. Green carnations are just one more bad thing about St. Patrick's Day.

Rules of green thumb. Bonsai trees are creepy-looking freaks of artifice more appropriate to a *Twilight Zone* set than a loved one's coffee table (plus they're very expensive) . . . Poinsettias are for business offices and parents only . . . Never dictate long or romantic messages to be written on a card enclosed with your flowers; even if the florist manages by some miracle to get it exactly right, the most poetic sentiment will, penned in another's hand, come across like once-chewed gum . . . Don't shy away from a bunch of daisies just because they're (usually) cheap; nothing is happier than a daisy . . . Geraniums may help keep away mosquitoes, but they don't make a very classy gift . . . Never give a cactus plant without thinking twice.

"My Love is like a red, red rose . . ." Burns was right, and just because you eschew clichés doesn't mean you have to throw out the baby with the bathwater. Hell, we're talking *National Flower* here. The dark-red ones should probably be reserved for dead gangsters, but there are upwards of 20,000 other varieties to choose from, and the woman of your dreams is not likely to despise you for sending her a dozen of any one of them. At least not the first few hundred times you do it.

FORMS OF ADDRESS

S todgy as it may seem in an age when the more rigid rules of etiquette have given way to simple common sense, we think first-naming has gotten out of hand, and not just when meeting someone for the first time (see INTRO-DUCTIONS).

Consider: People trying to sell you a product or service seem convinced that they have a leg up if they bypass the Mister stage altogether and immediately cuddle into a first-name basis. We say instant familiarity in pursuit of a sale is offensive (not to mention counterproductive). And what of the professional—typically a physician, frequently an attorney—who calls you by your first name but never encourages you to respond in kind? We say they're confusing professional status with social hierarchy.

Even worse, premature first-namers often presume to assign a diminutive when none is used by even your most intimate friends. Not every Richard is a Dick, after all, nor every William a Bill.

What can you do to discourage this? Unfortunately, not much. The buoyant salesman who first-names you after a much too hearty handshake is not the sort to get the point when you pointedly "Mister" him in response. And you don't want to suggest a more appropriate form of address to a doctor poking around on your corpus or a dentist armed with a sharp weapon.

You can, of course, set a good example by erring on the side of formality in dealing with people outside a clearly social setting. Stick with Mr., Mrs. (if you're sure that's what she prefers), and Ms. It's always easy to go from there to first names, but embarrassing and awkward to have to go the other way.

Postscript. All the classic etiquette books provide a list of proper forms of addresses to be used for certain titled personages. If you should be granted an audience with the Pope or the Prince of Wales, spend some time at the library before you go.

FRIENDLY WAGER

There's a big difference between a ten-dollar bet with your best friend on the Super Bowl and a ten-dollar bet on your regular Thursday-night squash game. And if you don't pay attention to that difference, you're in danger of letting a "friendly" wager damage your friendship.

When you bet the Celtics over the Lakers, or take the Royals and the odds over the Cardinals, the outcome of the wager is dependent on what a bunch of other guys do. If the bet is on competition between you and your friend, it can affect the outcome of the game.

It's not because of the size of the bet—presumably you both have the good sense to keep the amount low enough to be considered trivial as money. Nor is the danger that the bet will make you play any differently—presumably you both already play as hard as you can.

The real danger is that the wager, however small, is a gratuitous reminder of defeat. It creates, ever so slightly, a winner-loser relationship between two friends whose friendship is predicated on equality of status. Obviously the danger is lessened if you're evenly matched and each of you wins about half the time. And, just as obviously, it's increased if one of you tends to win the lion's share of your matches.

We're not saying you shouldn't make a harmless five-dollar bet with a friend now and then. We're saying you should be aware of what's going on so you can make sure it stays harmless. Otherwise the stakes of a "friendly wager" may be higher than you think.

GIFTS

It's better to give than to receive. It's the thought that counts. You shouldn't have. Money can't buy me love. . . .

And that's not the half of it. The giving and receiving of gifts is one of the most complicated and emotional interactions that we mortals must endure on a pretty regular basis—and often in public, no less. The way in which we react to the strain of exchanging gifts can be very telling indeed. Some people enjoy buying gifts for their loved ones; others respond by getting anxious, cranky, even paralyzed. We aren't psychiatrists here, so we wouldn't dream of trying to get at the psycho-emotional root of any problem you might have with picking out presents. We're just here to get you through it.

CHRISTMAS GIFTS

It's like talking about the weather. Everyone knows that Christmas is too commercial, but nobody is doing anything about it. Besides, what can you do? If you take a stand and declare a moratorium on all gifts, you may feel morally upright for a few moments, but sooner or later you'll realize that people just think you're too cheap and thoughtless to spring for a present. And if you decide to spend the money on a good cause—by donating money in their names to the Environmental Protection Agency or the Sylvester Stallone Fan Club—they'll think you've lost your mind. If you make it a policy to leave town for the holidays to avoid the whole thing, you could end up feeling tan but rotten.

Look at it this way: If you do continue to play the role of Scrooge, chances are that one of these days you won't have any friends to buy presents for.

So do yourself a favor and take a stand on something else (but not Valentine's Day) and try to look upon traditional holidays as opportunities to give tangible evidence of your feelings about your friends and family. We're not saying you'll ever learn to love it, but you could learn to hate it a little less.

To make Christmas shopping easier, try spreading the joy throughout the year, buying from catalogs, picking up a few small things when you travel, going with an inspiration, even if it occurs in August. It's acceptable to ask people what they'd like for Christmas, but the roundabout approach—asking close friends, for instance, or doing a little investigative research the next time you visit—is classier and more thoughtful. All-purpose gifts (a vase, a bottle of Scotch, a fruitcake) are better than none, but the true gift-giving spirit calls for the personal touch.

BIRTHDAY GIFTS

Birthdays are trickier than holidays, and not just because you don't get the day off from work and there isn't a window display at the mall to remind you of the Big Day. Some adults ignore their birthdays and don't care to be reminded of them, especially with ugly ties or gaudy costume jewelry. Others are disappointed when they don't receive at least a modest tribute at New York's Lincoln Center. The challenge is to discover which of your friends fall into which camp—and then to determine whether a birthday gift is in order.

Some sort of present is generally called for if you are seeing the birthday boy or girl on the Big Day, especially at an official birthday party. If it is a group affair, keep in mind that everyone is going to see the gift, so joke gifts should be tasteful, and more intimate offerings should wait until you've got some privacy.

P.S. Always remember your mother's birthday.

ANNIVERSARY GIFTS

When we think about anniversaries, we usually think about wedding anniversaries, and usually our own. One school of thought maintains that men give anniversary presents but don't as a rule receive them, but that strikes us as pre-feminist claptrap, not to mention a real gyp when it comes time to open packages. But don't worry about that for the moment.

Christmas and birthday gifts may come and go—clothes, perfume, a box of candy, a bottle of vintage champagne—but it's always seemed to us that an anniversary gift to a loved one should be one that lasts: crystal, jewelry, paintings, sculpture, photographs, small islands, etc. If you're an old-fashioned boy, you may want to dig up one of the old anniversary gift lists (paper for the first year, silver for the twenty-fifth, gold for the fiftieth, and lots of strangeness in between), but most people won't even know what you're talking about, and you'll end up having to explain your gift. Much better if you give some thought—lots—to your choice. If you're thinking about a small appliance, keep thinking.

Since wedding anniversaries are nothing if not personal, other people's anniversaries aren't really any of your business, and it's not usually appropriate to give gifts on those occasions. However, if you're invited to an anniversary party, it is thoughtful (but not mandatory) to take along a small gift for the happy couple.

DANGEROUS GIFTS

No matter how hard you try and how much thought you give to selecting a gift, there will be times when you make a mistake—when you give somebody something he or she doesn't like. If this happens to you rather a lot, there may be a message here for you. Perhaps you've been doing your shopping in the wrong part of the store.

Some gifts are safe—books, records, a piece of china, season tickets, fine glassware, vintage port, gift certificates, and lots more—but others can spell trouble. Unless you're very sure of your footing, beware of clothing, jewelry, paintings, sculpture, or anything else that is supposed to be displayed or worn.

(See also BREAD-AND-BUTTER GIFTS, SHOPPING, CHRISTMAS CARDS, MOTHER'S DAY, FATHER'S DAY, and VALENTINE'S DAY.)

"GIRLFRIEND"

S o there's this person of the female persuasion with whom you've been keeping regular company. You're not exactly planning to get married, and you may or may not be living together, but you're definitely an item. How can this, which sounds a lot like the answer to your prayers, be a problem? Well, you might ask. It's not, at least not usually. But every once in a while, at a party or a family gathering or a business dinner, when the time comes for you to introduce your companion, you find yourself literally at a loss for words.

"This is Catherine Deneuve, my ———" And then you clutch. What do you call her? Referring to her as "my friend" seems a little wimpy, "lady friend" is phony unless you're in a Noel Coward play, "lover" is way too sexual, "roommate" is too coy, and "main squeeze" is completely inappropriate unless she's Molly Ringwald and you're on your way to the homecoming game. Best to say nothing after her name. If she really is Catherine Deneuve, that will be enough.

When she's not around, you can call this lucky person your "girlfriend," despite the fact that under normal circumstances there is no such thing as a "girl" over 21. It's far from perfect, but it'll do.

One good reason to get engaged and/or married: "Fiancée" and "wife" may be old-fashioned words, but they sure make going to parties a lot easier.

GREASING A PALM

T he act of greasing someone's palm can be every bit as distasteful as it sounds. But sometimes a man has to do what he has to do, so you might as well learn how to do it right.

Fortunately, there's not a *lot* to learn about the subject. Just three rules: (1) Be discreet; (2) Don't even try unless there's a reasonable chance of success; and (3) Fold bills into neat little rectangles (the better to be palmed, then pocketed by their recipients).

Even if you're feeling like Frank Sinatra and believe the world should turn cartwheels to let you have everything your way, don't barge to the front of a line at a popular club brandishing a roll of bills. It may work if you're prepared to part with enough of them, but you'll also have to live with the stigma of having behaved (but never sung) like the Chairman of the Board.

Instead, step forward to the thug guarding the door, and as you tell him your name and the number in your party, make eye contact with the dead politician on the folded bill you're holding at your side. If you suspect the doorman may not be up on his American history, make sure he can see the number in the corner of the bill as well. At times like this, Andy Jackson is a much better president than Abe Lincoln.

Unlike a club, a restaurant has a finite capacity, so it's a bit harder getting a table at a chic place when you have neither reservation nor celebrity going for you. Harder, but not impossible.

Hand the maître d'hôtel your personal card when he greets you with his "No way, José" look, explain quietly that you have no reservation, but indicate that you and your companion(s) will be pleased to wait at the bar if it might be within his power to secure you a table in 15 minutes or so. The quarter hour gives him time to juggle his reservation list; the folded bill under your card gives him the incentive.

If he's a straight shooter and there's simply no hope, he'll return the card and the bill with his regrets. If he keeps both, the grace period for delivering the table is 15 minutes beyond the 15 you agreed to wait. But keep in mind that you have no recourse if he decides to stiff you or keep you waiting until you've drunk your appetite under the table. He's confident that you won't say, "Say, there, you scoundrel—return my bribe or get me a table!" And if you do, this kind of hard case is perfectly capable of staring you down as though you were a form of vermin the public health inspector missed in his last sweep through the kitchen.

At sports events—the other likely venue for palm greasing— the results are more predictable and the surcharge less onerous. If the ball park or arena is sold out, there's no way you are going to move down from nosebleed country short of dealing with a scalper. But if the stands are, say, half full at game time, your chances for getting closer for a small investment are good.

Walk up to the usher and hand him your crummy tickets, along with a bill folded and discreetly hidden, and a request for assistance in finding seats in his section. The more seats he has to find, the bigger the bill should be. And it's no use arguing if he says he can't help you: A good usher always knows which season boxes are likely to be empty, which ticket holders habitually come late, and where unfilled house seats are located.

Always make your approach from the proper entrance, as if you were just arriving and had tickets for that section. His bosses have minions with binoculars up in the rafters trying to catch ushers doing precisely what you're asking him to do. As it could mean his job if he's caught, he's much more likely to cold shoulder you if you come to his aisle directly from the cheap seats.

How much is enough? You'll have to learn by doing, and your education could be costly. Try two dollars a ticket at a sporting event, five dollars and up at a chic restaurant or club. How far up of course depends on the hotness of the spot.

Grooming

If you haven't already been told that every day you should take a shower, shave, clean your nails, brush your teeth, use a deodorant, and change your shirt, underwear, and socks, allow us to do the honors. Your wit and personality can take it from there. Of course those are just the basics. There's plenty more that the well-groomed man can and probably should do to make a nice appearance.

One of the greatest questions of our time is, Can a man who gets a professional pedicure be taken seriously? The answer, of course, is no. But what about manicures and massages and facials and tanning salons and cosmetic surgery? What indeed.

HAIR

Sure, you get it cut regularly, perhaps even by someone wearing spurs and four earrings in each ear. That's as it should be. But can a guy who goes beyond that to have his hair moussed, streaked, or permed really be regarded with a straight face? Should he allow complete strangers to tamper with his beard and mustache? Should he cover up a little gray? Should he wear a rug?

In these and all determinations we try to be realistic—times are, after all, changing—but we can't help but think that the fewer chemical changes your hair undergoes, the better, and that anything that makes you nervous about taking a shower with a lady can't be all good.

It's probably a mistake to streak, bleach, or color your hair. Have a permanent or body wave only if you're about to change jobs and move to another state. (Consider the plight of Earl Weaver, who tried out his new look on national TV.) And there's no such thing as a rug that doesn't look like one at least some of the time.

COLOGNE

Call it after-shave, call it skin bracer, call it cologne. We call it dangerous. And we also don't think it should be used as a substitute for a daily shower.

Things have loosened up a lot in the last few years, but even the least conservative guys still think that it's a mistake for a man's scent to precede him into a room. If you're sure that no one more than a few feet away will notice the cologne you're partial to, go ahead and slap it on. If you're unsure, give the stuff away.

COSMETICS

Use any kind of soap you fancy, fill your medicine cabinet to the rafters with astringent, moisturizers, and emery boards if you feel like it. But don't even think about wearing makeup unless you're about to go on *The Today Show*. The well-dressed man does not have a makeup line.

OTHER

Manicures are by no means required, but clean nails are, as surely as are sparkling teeth and fresh breath.

HANDSHAKE

A simple handshake tells you a lot about a man. For one thing, it tells you that he's probably an American. Europeans hug when they meet, the English nod, the Japanese bow, but Americans shake hands. And that's the way it is.

Extending an empty hand to show that you have no weapon, grasping another's hand to signify your human bond—you have to admit the handshake has impeccable symbolic credentials. Too bad that it has become so commonplace as to have lost most of its original meaning. Anyway, it's our way of saying hello, so we might as well get straight, once and for all, on the various kinds of handshakes, especially the only one that is correct.

The Politician's Pump. A familiar face with a toothy grin materializes out of a crowd as its owner grabs your right hand in a firm grip while simultaneously seizing your right forearm in his left hand. Two short, strong shakes and you find yourself being moved sideways as Teeth swivels to mug the next voter. (This is known as the Receiving Line Two-Hand when practiced by college presidents.)

The Preemptive Squeeze. All fingers and thumb. Your extended hand is caught just short of its target by a set of pincers that encloses your four fingers at the second knuckle and leaves your thumb pointing west. No palm contact whatsoever. One quick squeeze, a side-to-side waggle release, and your hand is unceremoniously dropped, leaving it utterly frustrated.

The Limp Fish. The most hated of all. Someone puts his fingers in your hand and leaves them there. Excusable in foreigners, who are still grappling with a language where "gh" and "f" sound alike (as in "tough fish"). For others, unacceptable.

The Macho Man. The old bone-crusher, the familiar signature of the emotionally insecure but physically strong. If you're alert, you can see this one coming in time to take countermeasures. The best defense is a good offense: Grab his hand toward the base of the palm to cut down on his fingers' leverage, and start your grip before he starts his. Of course, if he's strong enough and macho enough, it won't work, and he'll bond your individual digits into a single flipper for trying to thwart him.

The Preacher's Clasp. As your right hands join, his left folds over the top and immobilizes them both. Always accompanied by steady eye contact (no way you won't be the first to blink), and usually by a monologue delivered two inches closer to your face than is really necessary. Once the exclusive province of Presbyterian ministers, the Clasp is now practiced by a broad spectrum of the relentlessly sincere, including motivational speakers and honors graduates of weekend therapy marathons. The worst thing about it is that it makes your hand sweat.

The Right Way. A firm, full-handed grip, a steady squeeze, and a definite but understated downward snap (but no up-and-down pumping unless you're contemplating a disabling karate move), followed at once by a decisive release. Sounds easy enough, but how frequently do you encounter a really good one?

Shaking Hands with Women. No difference in grip (the Right Way is always right), but convention has it that you should wait for her to extend her hand first. These days, chances are good that she will.

Helping Her . . .

. . . ON/OFF TRAINS/BUSES

A man should always precede a woman off a bus or train so that he can turn back to offer a helping hand. Reverse positions when getting on—you hold back ready to catch her should she slip and fall. That's the way it's always been, and there's no good reason for changing. This holds true of course only if you are accompanying the woman in question. If she's a stranger, it's every man for himself. Nothing looks dumber than a man lagging back while a dozen or so women he doesn't even know push their way onto a crowded bus, particularly if you're wedged in behind him. The overriding rule of transportation etiquette: Keep the traffic moving.

. . . DRESS FOR THE OCCASION

If you're bringing a date to a party at the home of your friends, and she doesn't know them, it's up to you to crack the dress code and brief her thoroughly, unless the nature of the event clearly dictates the proper attire. There's no need to sniff out what she ought to wear to a Sunday afternoon barbecue; if she can't handle that one, you'd better call in sick. But lots of social functions, particularly dinner parties, could call for anything from jeans to long dresses. "I don't know, you look great in everything" won't help her choose which outfit to don, so don't be crushed if she fails to melt at the compliment. The solution is simple: Ask your hostess how to advise your companion on appropriate attire. The best clue is what the hostess herself is going to wear. If you ferret out that nugget of information, your date is home free.

. . . LIGHT UP

If you smoke, tobacco etiquette requires that you light a fire under the nose—Russell Baker's great way of putting it—of any woman in reach who slips a cigarette between her lips.

But if you don't smoke, there's no earthly reason why you should be expected to light someone else's cigarette, even one in the mouth of a female, unless you're hanging out in a bar, pretending to be Humphrey Bogart. It was not always so. Once upon a time a man was expected to carry a cigarette lighter on his person at all times on the odd chance that he might somewhere spot a woman with an unlit Chesterfield dangling from her lips. No matter that he wasn't a smoker himself; it was his duty always to be prepared to help her light up. The presumption apparently was that fair damsel could handle smoke but not fire. Nowadays we see that for what it is—foolishness. Vegetarians don't carry pork chops around in their pockets on the odd chance that a friend might have a hunger pang. If you don't smoke, and if you're not going on a camping trip, you don't need a lighter. If she can lift a cigarette, she can lift a match.

. . . INTO A TAXI

You open the taxi door, gallantly step aside, and offer your arm as she gets in first, right? Not necessarily. Depending on how she's dressed, it may make sense for you to go first. If you climb in first, you save her from having to slide over the hump in the floor, and from having to hike up her skirt, and from running the risk of of snagging a high heel in the process. You don't just shove your way past her, of course; you say something like, "It may be easier for me to go first." She'll have to close the door, it's true, but you can make up for it by paying the fare.

. . . PUT ON HER COAT

Old rules should never be discarded merely because they are old. Helping your female companion on with her coat looks right and feels good, so do it. One tip: If you're taller than she is, make sure you hold the coat at her shoulder height, not yours. Nothing looks sillier than a glamorously dressed woman jumping backward with arms thrusting blindly at the armholes of her coat. Here's the way to do it gracefully: Take the coat in both hands, rest your left hand on her left shoulder, dip your right hand slightly, and open the garment wide so she can put her right arm into the armhole without looking like a startled goose trying to take flight.

. . . SIT DOWN

Admit it: Just about every time you've held a chair for someone, the temptation has flashed through your mind, so fast as to be virtually subliminal, to pull the chair back at the last critical second. But since you are too much of a gentleman to go for a cheap laugh at someone else's expense (you *are,* aren't you?), you always resist that wicked impulse. Even so, it doesn't always go smoothly, and occasionally becomes a near fiasco in which you risk being charged for assault with a deadly chair. Worry no more; help is here.

Like parallel parking, helping a woman sit down at a dinner table should be accomplished in three precise moves, no matter how tight the fit. First, pull the chair away from the table far enough for her to step in front of it easily. Second, as she starts her downward move, ease the chair forward *part* of the way (but not so far that the front of the chair bangs her behind the knees). Third, once her derrière is in place, make any final adjustment needed to get her close enough to the table. She will signal this final fine-tuning by lifting herself ever so slightly while you push.

If that seems like a lot of explaining for so slight an act, well, it is. But good form in social behavior consists of informed attention to detail, and performing small deeds of this sort gracefully sets you apart from the crowd.

On the other hand it really would be funny, just once, and only if she were someone really pompous who needed to be brought down a peg or two, and if you could be absolutely sure she wouldn't hurt herself (the kind who deserves it is also the kind who sues at the drop of a hat), it really would be funny to . . .

. . . CARRY STUFF

Carrying her books home from school might have been a great way to impress girls when Mickey Rooney and Judy Garland made up the first Brat Pack, but nowadays you should think twice before grabbing a woman's heavy stuff with a hearty, "Here, let me help you with that!" The problem with such an approach is that it is unwittingly patronizing and carries with it all sorts of implicit assumptions about her fragility, her weakness, and her inability to fend for herself. Would you grab heavy stuff away from another man without asking if he needed help with his load? Of course not, and so it should be with a woman.

"May I help you with that?" is the question you ask. And don't let your manly feelings get hurt if her answer is, "Thanks, I can manage."

How Old Are You?

I t's a funny thing about age—it matters to the most peculiar people at the most unpredictable times. And believe it or not, it will eventually matter (possibly a lot) to you. One introspective man we know said that he knew he was getting old when he realized that he would be embarrassed, and possibly arrested, if he dated a girl in her teens. Have no doubt—your epiphany is coming.

Even if you're not hung up about being usurped by the next generation, you are bound to be surrounded by people who are. Be careful, just in case. Traditions come and go, and even though Jane Fonda and Linda Evans have made it downright fashionable to be over forty, it's still not appropriate to ask a lady her age. And it never will be.

However, if you've absolutely got to know how old a woman is, there are ways of finding out, and we're not talking about rifling her wallet while she's out of the room. For instance, a discussion of Kennedy's assassination can dampen the mood, but once one gets started, people are almost physically compelled to tell what they were doing when they heard the news. If she says she was so upset that she colored outside the lines when her mom read her the headline, you've got a general idea. Or if she's a basketball fan who went to UCLA, find out whether she cheered her head off for Bill Walton or Walt Hazzard. Other points of reference: Woodstock, *The Mary Tyler Moore Show,* and "Yellow Submarine." Use your imagination, but be subtle.

What you do with this information once you've got it is up to you. Dating out of your age group is quite common these days, but it does leave you open to ridicule, and sometimes scorn, by the more Neanderthal of your acquaintances.

The sooner you come to grips with telling people the truth about your own age, the better off you'll be. It's far too complicated to lie, anyhow (see NANCY REAGAN), so you might as well come clean.

HOUSEWORK

The last thing in the world a guy needs is dishpan hands, but he also doesn't need a visit from the Board of Health. And *somebody* has to clean up this mess. Ideally, of course, it will be somebody else. The sooner you can afford to pay someone to handle the maintenance of your apartment, the better (see CLEANING HELP). Get a part-time job or sell the watch you got when you graduated from college.

But until you've got thirty or so bucks a week to spare, learn how to cope with no-wax floors as best you can and try to keep the bathtub clean while maintaining your self-respect. Don't wear rubber gloves, at least not in front of anyone. The next thing you know, you'll be thinking about putting on a hair net while you cook. And remember the most important rule of housework: If you clear off enough surfaces (and we're too fastidious to speculate about how you do it), at least the place will *look* clean.

All this wisdom applies if you're responsible for the cleanliness of your own place. If you share quarters with someone else, there are—naturally—a few wrinkles. If life were perfect, household chores would fall to those who don't mind doing them, and by some miracle you and your apartment mate wouldn't mind doing exactly 50 percent of the work. But life's not perfect, and we've never met anyone who likes cleaning the bathroom.

So the easiest way to spread the wealth is to write each chore on a piece of paper and put the pieces in piles of ascending drudgery. You'll probably have at least three stacks—of perfectly acceptable, not-too-terrible, and absolutely awful tasks. Using the mathematical skills you learned back in fourth grade, divide the piles until you've each got an equal burden. To make matters even fairer, switch off regularly.

If you have no idea of where to start when it comes to housework, here's a list to get you going:

1. Chores that should be done every day. Nothing, really. (And you were worried!) Some people say that it should be a law

to make your bed every day, but we don't agree. However, we do think you should make your bed if there's even a slim chance that someone besides you is going to see it.

2. Chores that should be done every couple of days. Wash the dishes, take out the trash, and hang up your clothes.

3. Chores that should be done once a week. Dust, vacuum, clean the bathtub and toilet, and replace your sheets and towels.

4. Chores that should be done every couple of weeks. Deal with the laundry and give the furniture a quick once-over with spray polish.

5. Chores that should be done once a month. Wash the floors and possibly the windows.

6. Chores that should be done every few months. Defrost the refrigerator and clean the oven.

But we still say that your best bet is still to skip a few meals and hire help.

(See also CLEANING HELP, COHABITATION, and ROOMMATE.)

HOST

Being a host means lots of things. It means being in charge. It means always thinking first of the well-being of your guests. It means anticipating, planning, executing. It means that you can never relax entirely, or drink as much as you'd like, or go to bed early with a good book.

All of this may sound like a superhuman sacrifice, but the fact is that hosting a successful dinner party, or cocktail party, or poker game, or fishing weekend, or whatever, can be one of the most generous and most satisfying things you can do for the people you care about. It may be tiring, but your efforts will be appreciated.

The basics of being a host involve choosing and orchestrating the event and picking up the tab, but there are countless variations on this theme. Most people entertain over meals in their home, but many single men don't enjoy that. There's no rule that says you can't have a few laughs when you're showing others a good time. You'll have the best time if you do what comes naturally, whether it's doing a mean imitation of Craig Clairborne in the kitchen or buying a dozen box seats and springing for hot dogs and beer at the ball park or arranging two or three foursomes and a surf-and-turf dinner at the country club. Being a host is not a question of cash outlay or extravagance. It's a state of mind.

If one of your guests offers to contribute his or her famous guacamole or cheesecake or brownies or party tapes, don't feel you must accept, but don't automatically say no either. Even a perfect host can use a little help from his friends once in a while.

(See also INVITATIONS, DINNER PARTY, COCKTAIL PARTIES, BREAD-AND-BUTTER GIFTS, and WEEKEND GUEST.)

Introductions

Etiquette gurus make a fair to-do about introductions, and for good reason. The way you introduce yourself to another person, or introduce two other persons to each other, is the very first step in something brand new and laden with potential and mystery, however brief the encounter might turn out to be. At least that's the way you should approach the act of bringing two people together.

Tradition says that you should introduce the younger person to the older, if both are of the same sex, and the male to the female, if they are not. Tradition is right, to a point. But you don't have to check IDs to make sure of comparative ages before getting on with names, and sometimes it's more sensible (and will seem more courteous) to introduce the person you know less well to the person you know better, regardless of age, sex, or national origin.

It's often appropriate, and always helpful, to add a little something to the names to give the newlymets a bit of common ground for conversation. Do not, however, identify someone by what he or she does for a living. Someone who is a poet at heart does not necessarily want to be identified as a dentist, even if he does drill teeth to pay the rent. And saddling someone with a professional mug sheet might set up an artificial barrier with the party of the second part. (Nobody likes lawyers, for instance, so identifying your friend Jane as one may make it harder for your friend Dick to recognize her many fine qualities.)

Now the tough part: What do you do when you start to introduce two people and your mind suddenly goes blank when it comes to their names? Punt. What else can you do? This is one of the most frequent sources of embarrassment in polite society. And when it happens, you live in constant dread that it will happen again—which only makes it more likely that it will. If you've known the person whose name has just slipped your mind since kindergarten, you can make a joke of it, complete with reference to

Freud. But if the nameless person is an acquaintance whose name you should remember but don't, you're in trouble.

Don't expect to find a satisfactory solution here. We deal in social behavior, not miracles. You can, if you recognize before you start to speak that you've forgotten a person's name, simply skip the introduction altogether and start talking about something else. This should prompt one person to offer his or her name, and that will nudge the other to respond in kind. *Then* you can say, "Oh—I thought you two knew each other," and you're off the hook.

That won't always work, of course, and you'll be left with nothing to do but apologize and have to ask the person his or her name. Resist the tendency to *over*-apologize. The misdeed is done, and saying you are sorry a thousand different ways only calls more attention to your gaffe. Follow the lead of the ace relief pitcher who gives up a ninth-inning home run to lose the game: Let it go and look ahead to tomorrow.

If you're the one being introduced, always be prepared to jump in and help in the event that the person making the introductions forgets *your* name. This is both an act of mercy for the poor soul who would otherwise be left groping blindly in an empty memory bank and pure self-interest—you do want the person you're meeting to know who you are, after all.

First-name introductions are for fern bars. Anywhere else, give your whole name when meeting someone for the first time, even if your surname abounds in syllables and consonants and has to be repeated twice. If a third party handles the introductions and shorts you half a moniker—"Jack, I want you to meet Jill"—finish the job with a "Hello, I'm Jack Spratt." The practical reason for using both names—so she can find your name in the telephone book later—is less critical here than what you project about yourself by your choice. First-naming suggests superficiality, lack of seriousness, and immaturity. Grown-ups use both names.

INVITATIONS

Some of the pleasantest of all social occasions are those that happen serendipitously, but (alas) most parties and such require planning. And planning means, among many other things, extending and receiving invitations.

RECEIVING THEM

It's been said a million times, so once more won't hurt: When you're invited to something and asked to respond, protocol dictates that you do so—promptly. That means if someone calls you on the phone, say yes or no right then, if you can. Positive responses are easy ("That sounds wonderful. I'd love to be there"), but turning somebody down can be hard, especially if you're saying no because you just don't want to go. Try, "That sounds great, but I'm afraid I can't make it. I've got other plans, though I really appreciate your asking me." You don't have to explain yourself any further (e.g., "That was the weekend I was planning to take my wide ties in to be narrowed"), and if somebody is rude enough to press you for an explanation, be vague. Say you've got family or business commitments. If you're up against the wall, drop broad hints about major surgery. It'll serve the person right.

If you can't give an immediate answer, explain that you have to check with your wife, your schedule, your astrologer, your nutritionist, or whatever and ask if it would be all right if you called later that day/tomorrow/Wednesday. If you really do need until Wednesday but your prospective host doesn't like the idea of waiting, say, "Then perhaps I'd better say no. I don't want to hold you up or upset your plans." No hard feelings on either side. If you do get the reprieve you ask for, be sure to call promptly on the day you said you would. Don't make your host call you.

By the way, if you aren't asked to bring a date, that means you're not supposed to. If you've got a girlfriend (see "GIRLFRIEND") whom your host doesn't know about, and your days of going to parties stag are over, it's perfectly all right to say so and ask if it would be all right if she accompanied you. It's also perfectly all right (but a little tacky unless it's an intimate dinner party) for the host to say no.

SENDING THEM

The world seems to be divided into those people who give parties and those who don't. If you're in the second group but want to take a stab at joining the first, you'll have to learn to cope with the invitation.

There are two kinds—oral and written. Formal occasions (presidential inaugurations, weddings, etc.) demand something white, tasteful, and professionally printed, and it's usually more efficient (and more festive) to send informal invitations to large parties through the mail. The lead time depends on the event; wedding invitations usually go out six weeks ahead; for other parties three weeks will do nicely.

The most important thing to know about written invitations is that despite the fact that RSVP is written on them as big as life and that up until now you thought your friends were a thoughtful, polite, swell group of people, you might not get responses from as many as half of the people you invite. The challenge to which you must rise is to find out who is coming without ending up thinking that all of your friends are complete swine.

Give people until a week before the event and then start calling them on the phone. It's a drag, but it's got to be done. (Remember this feeling the next time you get an invitation.)

For relatively small gatherings it's customary to do your inviting by phone (about two weeks in advance, perhaps less), but that can also get complicated—for instance, when you start with a date you like and a guest list of eight compatible people, and you end up with three yesses, three nos, and a couple of maybes. Be firm with the maybes—give them a couple of days to get back to you and follow up. If your guests' schedules are just too complicated to make this particular party work on this particular date, it's perfectly all right to call it off and reschedule.

RECIPROCATING

Think twice before accepting an invitation to dinner at the home of someone whose company you don't enjoy, because if you go, sooner or later you'll have to have him or her back. If the friendship is doomed, you may as well nip it in the bud.

Reciprocating doesn't necessarily mean reciprocating in kind, though. That's why the cocktail party was invented—so you can entertain on a grand scale even if you're not a great cook and/or made of money. And restaurants were invented so that you could throw a dinner party even if you don't have a hot plate, let alone a formal dining room with a dimmer switch. The general rule is an eye for an eye and a dinner for a dinner, but there are lots of exceptions.

(See also DINNER PARTY, COCKTAIL PARTIES, and RSVP.)

JEWELRY

Some hard-liners say that the only jewelry a man should wear is a watch, cuff links that run absolutely no risk of becoming a conversation piece and, with black tie, studs. However, because we like to be men of the people, we're prepared to accept tie clips and pins—not too flashy, if you please—and a ring, so long as it's not worn on the pinky. (Ideally it would be a signet ring that belonged to your grandfather, the Earl.) Forget gold chains.

Somebody once said that a *woman* should be the showcase of a man's wealth. Words to live by.

JOKES

If God had meant for all of us to be funny, he would have given all of us baggy pants and seltzer bottles and an arrow through our heads. But Noooo! He bestowed the gift of really good joke-telling on only a precious few.

Even though the telling of jokes is one of the trickiest skills around—for every belly laugh a raconteur produces, there are a dozen frozen stares—we continue to give it a try and we probably always will. It can serve to relieve tension, and it sometimes helps break the ice. So, okay, go ahead and tell a joke now and then if you must. And when you're with your near and dear friends, feel free to take a few chances and make a fool of yourself. But when you're among strangers, take our advice. Please.

• Telling jokes to people you don't know can be very chancy. Unless you've got a never-fail joke that you're positive that no one has ever heard, fight the feeling.

• Avoid jokes that involve race, religion, ethnic groups, or sex (no easy feat, to be sure). That includes the one about the one-legged belly dancer and the traveling salesman.

• If you can't stand it anymore, go ahead, tell your joke. But make sure it's short, pertinent, and doesn't make anyone feel stupid. Whenever possible, avoid accents.

• If someone else starts a joke, don't interrupt, and when he's finished, just laugh politely. Don't try to top him even if you can.

KISSING

A kiss, by definition, is an intimate act. Call us old-fashioned, but we think it should, for the most part, take place in private. Oh, sure, joyful greetings at airports can be accompanied by a public kiss, and celebrations at weddings and birthdays and reunions are appropriate occasions for kissing in front of strangers, and New Year's Eve wouldn't be the same without kisses at midnight, and—well, come to think of it, maybe there are a lot of instances when a kiss is a perfectly acceptable, even a preferred form of public interaction between a man and a woman.

But it should be clear that what we're talking about here is the kiss as an expression of affection, not of passion. There is a difference, and two people locked in an embrace on a busy street corner are practically insisting that passersby invade their privacy. Maybe this is how to draw the line: A public kiss should not be mistaken for foreplay.

Europeans, and particularly the French and Italians, are notorious public kissers, if you can call the pecks they deliver to both cheeks kisses. Keep this in mind the next time you are in Monaco. But remember: Just because it looks suave at the baccarat tables does not mean you should try it back home at the water cooler. Kissing and business are a bad mix.

There is one form of "kissing" that you should do your best to eliminate from human interaction altogether. That is, of course, the current social custom of a man and a woman putting their cheeks together and kissing air. This not a fit way for consenting adults to handle hellos and goodbyes. The next time she offers you her cheek, kiss it square-on—or, better still, gently take her chin, swivel her face a few degrees, and plant one smack on her lips. Even in public.

LETTERS

The telephone has so completely supplanted the letter as a means of communication in our half of this century that you don't even hear people complaining anymore about the decline of letter writing as an art form. That's a pity, because there will always be something special about a letter.

On the other hand, the good side of our modern neglect of letter writing is that it gives you a golden opportunity to distinguish yourself. While others reach out and touch one another, albeit after 5:00 p.m. at a 30-percent discount, you can do something far more rare, and hence more valuable: You can write a letter.

We're talking now about a personal letter to a friend or family member, not a love letter (see LOVE LETTERS) or one of the notes required from time to time by specific social circumstances (see THANK YOU, CHRISTMAS CARDS, and RSVP) or a business letter (see some other book).

The only requirement of a letter is that it contain information of probable interest and/or importance to its recipient. Form, length, and style are entirely up to the writer. Unless you're writing to your high school English teacher, you won't go wrong if you pay heed to the old adage and "write like you talk," even if your grammar is a little shaky either way.

There are a few "don'ts" you should know about. Don't write a letter with the expectation of getting one in return, unless you get some kinky pleasure out of disappointment. Don't complain in your letter about how long it's been since you heard from the person you're writing to. And, unless you're still in graduate school and convinced that you're the only one in the world with no free time, don't ever, *ever* write one of those "Dear Friends and Family" letters that gets photocopied and sent to all the people you assume are waiting breathlessly for an update on your life.

A yellow legal pad is better than nothing, but good stationery is obviously in your future if you take a fancy to writing letters (see STATIONERY). And, even though the Emily Posts of the world will scream to high heaven, we say using a typewriter or word processor is okay if only because most of us don't study penmanship in school anymore. (But no letters of condolence in pica *or* elite, please.)

Any time is a good time for a letter, so long as you keep in mind that it will have the most impact when it is least expected. If you need an occasion to jump-start yourself into action, think about the nature and history of your friendship with the friend you're planning to write. Did you used to live and die together with the Bears on fall weekends? Then Super Bowl Week will always be a good time for a letter, even in years that Chicago doesn't make it that far.

You get the idea, but you really don't need it. After all, a letter to someone you care about doesn't require an occasion. Write on!

LIMOUSINES

Along, elegant limousine pulling up to a theater, restaurant, or club and disgorging its spiffily clad occupants almost inevitably ignites a spark of curiosity, a flash of glamour, perhaps a tinge of envy. No matter that the classy-looking vehicle is—99 percent of the time—on hire for the night and not drawn from anyone's personal stable of status symbols. Or that this ostentatious mode of transportation—hitherto associated with rock stars, princes of capitalism, deposed Latin American dictators living in exile, first-generation filthy rich, and those to the manner born—has become the conveyance of preference to high school proms in the nation's upwardly mobile suburbs. No, even among the most worldly and knowing of us, a limousine can still evoke glittering fantasies of opening night on Broadway or Oscar night in L.A.

All the more reason, the next time you plan a special night on the town, to treat yourself to a limo. Here are some things to consider:

• For starters, of course, don't refer to it as a limo. Call it a car. (Cool is part of the fantasy; live it.)

• Any occasion will do as an excuse. Going to City Hall to get married, transporting you and your pals to the Big Game, party-hopping during the holiday season—all can be accomplished as effectively in a station wagon, of course, but a limousine adds equal measures of class and comfort to the venture and instantly turns a trip into an event.

• Don't worry about having to skip lunch for the next three years to pay for it. A standard limo costs about $100 to $125 for four hours' minimum in most places. Not cheap, compared with the family Toyota, but less than you probably expected.

• Now, there are limos, and there are *limos* (or *cars,* if you've been paying attention). A bare-bones, off-the-rack, standard issue, no-frills limousine will haul you around in plenty of style. But a stretch à la mode—i.e., an oversized limousine whose fridge is stocked with champagne and caviar—is horsepower of a different color. Think of it as the difference between Atlantic City and Vegas.

- Big as it is, a limousine is not a bus. It *can* transport six people (three on the back seat, two on the jump seats, and one up front with the driver), but only at a considerable reduction in aura. Four is best.

- Limousine seats are lower and deeper than in standard sedans, so your assignment as the host is to help other passengers—male and female—get out (in is easy) without struggle. it goes without saying that the host sits on one of the jump seats. (Exception: Anyone over six feet two inches tall is going to look like Ichabod Crane and feel like a pretzel perched on a jump seat with knees at chin level. Use common sense.)

- The fellow behind the wheel is your *driver,* not your chauffeur (unless you buy the vehicle and hire him full-time), not one of the guys from the car pool, certainly not your dad. Don't be haughty, don't say funny things like "Home, James"—and don't include him in your party just because you're not accustomed to dealing with drivers.

- A service charge is always built into the rental fee, but give something above that directly to the driver—at least $10, more if the evening has been especially long or he has been especially helpful.

- Save it for the nighttime. There's something corrupt about riding in a limousine in the bright light of day, maybe because that's when they're most likely to contain diplomats and lords of industry instead of people having a good time.

When in doubt, remember this: With the possible exception of funerals, no trip that begins and end in a limousine can be all bad.

Liquor Cabinet

W e can't stop you from drinking Bellinis. After all, it's your life. We just don't think you have to serve them up at home. We're here to tell you about the magic potions with which a gentleman's liquor cabinet should be amply stocked.

Kir royales come and go, but some things never change. With beer, Scotch, bourbon, rum, vodka, gin, sweet and dry vermouth, sherry, brandy, and a few liqueurs on hand, you'll be the perfect host. Throw in seltzer, tonic, three or four kinds of fruit juice, an ice bucket, a cocktail shaker, a wine carafe, some mixed nuts, and *The Esquire Wine and Liquor Handbook,* and you can rule the world.

If you collect liquor samples from airplanes, you should be ashamed of yourself.

You'll also need glasses—tall ones for gin and tonic, short ones for bourbon on the rocks, liqueur glasses, and wineglasses. If you're feeling extravagant, add some champagne glasses just for the two of you, and keep in mind that a martini tastes twice as good in a proper martini glass.

(See also WINE.)

LIVING QUARTERS

You are not just what you eat. These days you are also how you decorate your apartment, even if it's your first one.

Everyone is entitled to enjoy a nice long period of decorating with orange crates and large cushions strewn around on the floor, but sooner or later you have to say goodbye to all that and give serious thought to having a grown-up place in which to live. We're not talking showplace here; we're talking about something that every woman who visits won't be *dying* to get her hands on. Ideally you'll begin to develop your own style as you gain a little decorating experience (and a lot of advice). These few guidelines should tide you over until you have the confidence to decorate on your own.

THE BASICS

For the living room you'll need a few basics: a couch, a rug, a coffee table, an end table, a couple of lamps, a chair or two, and a place to store books, records, and your TV. Remember, it's a living room, not just a stop on the way to the kitchen.

If you've got no color sense at all, keep in mind that you'll never be a laughing stock if you stay with earth tones. Shag carpeting is for the insecure; you're man enough for dhurries or some other thin rug. In your perfectly admirable desire to take the minimalist approach to decorating you may think that you want to leave the floors bare, but you really don't.

When you look for coffee tables, keep in mind that chrome and glass have to be polished every half hour, and strange shapes lose their appeal more quickly than you think. Go for a nice rectangle, big enough for a stack of magazines, a large bowl of popcorn, a pitcher of margaritas, and your feet.

Picking a chair is a little trickier. What do you go for, comfort or class? It's not necessary to go whole hog and get a Laz-E-Boy, but it's definitely important to find something that will be Your Chair. (Archie Bunker wasn't wrong about everything.) You don't want to read Proust or watch a seven-game series in anything but complete comfort. And while you're at it, there's nothing wrong with hassocks. Lamps are easy: The simpler the better—no exceptions. We're not optometrists, and we can never remember which shoulder a light should shine over anyhow, so ask questions and experiment with wattage and such.

If you haven't yet been introduced to the wonders of the Wall Unit, it's about time you learned. Ostensibly it's a place for you to put your books, your television, your radio, your tapes and cassettes, your tape deck, record player, and any other evidence of Eighties technology that you've managed to accumulate. Actually, if it's the kind that has cabinets with doors, it also gives you a place to throw your socks when you have unexpected company. And finally it helps you make one of the hardest decorating decisions that you'll ever face. When you have a Wall Unit, your stereo speakers go on either side of it.

THE BATHROOM

Bathrooms are boring, and it's a good idea to keep them that way. Go ahead and add a few homey touches, but don't be tempted to make your shower curtain the showpiece of your home. Buy nice fluffy towels that cost less than you spend on your shirts. Display your hair dryer if you must, but foot powder and hair spray should be your little secret. If you're stuck for a color scheme, you can always fall back on a nautical blue and white. Nobody cares much one way or the other unless it's not clean. Be sure it is.

THE BEDROOM

Bedrooms are less boring than bathrooms, but that doesn't mean that strangers passing through to leave their coats on your bed should find out too many facts about your personal life. Forget pinups and other holdovers from dorm life, but feel free to display pictures of yourself as captain of the track team or meeting Sammy Davis, Jr. Since most apartments don't have trophy rooms—more's the pity—bedrooms have to suffice as display areas for mementos.

Brass beds are classy; waterbeds are sexy; single beds are pitiful. Just about any kind of double bed is okay, but if you've got the room, go for a queen-size and make sure your sheets are mostly cotton and have as few flowers and small animals on them as possible. Bedspreads are fine, but don't forget about quilts and comforters. They feel good, and they do wonders when they're tossed on an unmade bed.

THE KITCHEN

Now for the kitchen. If you cook, it may well be your favorite room in the house, and you have very strong ideas about how it should look. If you don't cook, you probably don't much care how it looks. Basically you don't want to give the impression that you're the kind of fellow who alphabetizes the spices in his spice rack, but you're not looking to be Dustin Hoffman making French toast in *Kramer vs. Kramer* either. In short, you don't make your own yogurt, but you do make a mean pot of chili. (See COOKING).

Here are a few kitchen decorating hints for the non-cook:

• Hang pots and pans and large utensils on the wall or from the ceiling.

• Don't put cute magnetized animals on your refrigerator.

• Dust your stove once in a while.

• Remember the nine food groups: club soda, beer, wine, bourbon, popcorn, crackers, cheese, vanilla ice cream, and Hershey's chocolate syrup. Don't stay home without them.

ACCESSORIES

We've come a long way from bowling trophies, but chairs and lamps do not a cosy, friendly apartment make. In order to make the place you live in truly yours, you have to let your taste and personality show. Plants and flowers are always appropriate, but there are responsibilities attached to both. Plants have to be watered and sprayed, and flowers have to be arranged and then thrown out no more than a week after they're officially dead.

If you do decide to start some kind of collection and display it, arrange it on a table, not up on a shelf somewhere. Collecting is supposed to be fun. Two final suggestions: It shouldn't look as if you bought the whole collection at a tag sale last weekend, and it's a big mistake to collect things you don't really like. If your friends are as observant and thoughtful as we hope they are, you're going to be getting brass rubbings for your birthday for a long, long time.

ART

So you've got your tasteful couch and your favorite chair and your understated lamps. The bad news is that you have yet to face your most difficult decorating decision: What should you put on the walls to make the place look distinctive?

If you know about art and you know what you like, go for it. If you're fresh out of ideas, you can't go wrong with botanicals, Chagall prints, old quilts, and movie posters. Try one of each, and shell out a few bucks on frames while you're at it. It will seem like a lot of money, but it's well spent.

Photographs of family and friends are wonderful to have around, but they belong in the bedroom, not the living room. You're going to make new friends (and maybe even new family), and you don't want them to feel left out. To be on the safe side keep pictures of old girlfriends and former wives out of sight. There's no point in asking for trouble, especially in such a great-looking apartment!

(See also HOUSEWORK.)

LOCKER ROOM

H ere's a fact of nature that ranks right up there with Newton's Second Law of Thermodynamics as a constant in the universe: The best-hung guys are always the ones who spend the most time naked in locker rooms. If that's you, more power to you. The rest of us are going to have a little chat about locker-room manners.

Baseball players feel so strongly about the place where they change into their uniforms and shower after a game that they refer to it, always, as a clubhouse, never a locker room. You undoubtedly don't spend as much time hanging out before your regular Wednesday squash match as a major league ballplayer does before a game, but even the locker room of a big-city health club has its telling rituals and unspoken etiquette. And the posher the club, the more you will be expected to conform to those dos and don'ts, written and otherwise.

That's because the locker room is more than a place to stash clothes while you work up a sweat. It's a sanctuary, a place for escape. This is particularly so if it's part of a private sports club of some sort, but it's also true of the most egalitarian Y. And it means, first and foremost, that topics of conversation likely to cause tension and anxiety should be left outside the door.

The first among these is money. That wasn't a problem when we were teenagers, because young males in locker rooms talk almost exclusively about young females. ("Talk" is perhaps too passive a word; "scream" is more like it.) The opposite sex utterly dominated locker room exchange, clearly because sex always has been and—God willing—always will be the greatest single source of teenage anxiety.

Maybe it's a sign of growing up (or just growing older), but adult males don't talk about women in locker rooms nearly as much as they did when they were in high school, because most are too preoccupied with career and success to admit of any other abiding interest.

That's why Rule No. 1 of locker room etiquette is "Don't talk business," which is shorthand for "Don't introduce topics of conversation that might lead to stress or anxiety, either for you or for anyone in earshot." Talk about your new court shoes, about the game you just won (or lost), about the Raiders' chances this year. But don't talk bout how nervous you are about the firm's upcoming performance review, or whether the new tax law will kill your chances of getting a cabin at the lake, or which way that hot little biotech stock is going to go in the short term.

Talking about such matters in one of the few settings in this crazy world designed to insulate you from stress undermines your reason for being there in the first place. Worse still is the effect such chatter might have on innocent bystanders who overhear you, when all they were looking for was a little workout with the weight machines and a lot of peace of mind.

There are other things to keep in mind. Remember, for instance, that territoriality counts for more in confined spaces— that means keeping your stuff together and not spreading your gear out in front of other guys' lockers. Tipping attendants is usually a matter of club policy or common practice; it's your job to find out what that is. (This is not a good place to be cheap; word travels fast.) Your average locker room is no place for elaborate grooming rituals, so wax your mustache somewhere else. Keep family troubles out of the locker room. And, of course, you don't need to be reminded not to leave dirty, sweat-soaked gear in your locker until next Thursday's workout—do you?

But, above all, obey Rule No. 1. Help turn your locker room into a clubhouse.

LOVE LETTERS

I t's definitely better to have loved and lost than never to have loved at all. However, whether it's a great idea to put your feelings in writing is still subject to brisk debate. Logic notwithstanding, sometime or other in your life you will almost certainly be tempted to take pen in hand and spill your guts. If you're lucky, you'll get more than a few billets-doux in return.

WRITING THEM

God knows we presume a lot in these pages, but even we are not so arrogant as to tell you what you ought to say in a love letter. How do you love her? *You* count the ways. But be sure that you count them by hand (there's something about a dot-matrix printer that takes the romance out of things) on presentable stationery. Office stationery is absolutely out, but on rare occasions hotel/motel stuff works nicely. Among other things it suggests to the lucky recipient that (a) you were indeed where you said you were going to be, (b) you were alone in your room, and (c) that you were missing her too much to read the Bible or watch TV.

SAVING THEM

Only a certifiable lunatic keeps copies of the love letters he *writes*, so we'll concern ourselves here with what you should do with the ones you *get*, you dog, you. One school of thought says smile, sigh, thank your lucky stars, and pitch 'em—no ifs, ands, or buts. Why, these scholars ask, keep embarrassing evidence lying around in shoe boxes where anyone can get a look at them? After all, you never know who's going to go poking around in your sock drawer. This advice is sound in a paranoid sort of way, but it lacks a certain, shall we say, feeling.

The other school says that only a robot would toss away the heartfelt sentiments of a woman in love. Even if you haven't seen the lady in years, those letters are part of your history, like your high school yearbook and your Mamas and Papas albums and the scorecard for the first time you broke 100 without a single mulligan. And there's no use pretending that women are the only ones who are sentimental slobs about this sort of thing. If you do throw caution—and your love letters—to the winds, you may live to regret it.

(See also LETTERS and STATIONERY.)

LUNCH DATE

The key word here is "date." We're definitely not talking here about the business lunch, or grabbing a sandwich with some pals, and certainly not about "luncheon," which should be avoided like the plague. We're talking about a date, with a member of the opposite sex, as in boy-meets-girl, for lunch.

Why lunch? Well, mainly because it's the perfect solution for the dilemma of what-to-do, where-to-go, on a first date. It's not open-ended, but has a predetermined beginning and conclusion. It postpones (if you want it to) the question of sex (whether to have it, that is), and thus reduces tension. (Unless, of course, lunch is provided by room service.) It lets you say you have to be back at the office by 1:30, but then allows you to stay until 2:30 if you're having fun. And it costs less than an evening on the town. So what if the light is less flattering?

The trick is to pick the spot with care. Steer clear of places where you and the guys congregate for after-work beers, places that evoke fresh memories of old flames, and places where you're likely to run into ex-anythings. The ideal locale for a lunch date need not be a four-star establishment where everyone else is eating high on the expense account hog. But it shouldn't be a barbecue joint, either. Table cloths, *sí;* ketchup bottles on the table, no. You don't need an establishment with a sommelier, but you do need to be able to get a bottle of decent wine with your meal. You want salads, not salad bars.

In most cities the kind of place you're looking for will require a reservation. Often it will be ethnic, probably Italian. Just be sure that it goes light on the *Gemütlichkeit.* You never want to be in a place where the waiters suddenly burst into song, no matter whose birthday it is. And theme restaurants are even more frightful in the glare of day than they are at night—and the food's no better.

Lunch dates are also good for blind dates and for working through the early stages of a relationship. They're even good for breaking up when things go bad, although odds are you won't enjoy your linguini with clam sauce nearly as much as you normally do.

(See also BLIND DATE, BREAKING UP, DATING, and DINNER DATE.)

MANNERS ABROAD

Rich, loud, ignorant, boorish, insensitive, thoughtless, arrogant, overbearing. Blundering over hallowed standards of decorum in London, blustering through unfamiliar menus in Paris, complaining that no one understands him in Rome. Who else could we possibly be talking about but that storied figure, the American Abroad?

First the Peace Corps, then the wave of American student travelers since the mid-1960s did their part to put this stereotype to rest. But it has been painfully slow to die.

That's a pity, because it doesn't take much to be a courteous visitor. All you have to do is to remember that you are in someone else's hometown, and then behave the way you would prefer to have a stranger behave in yours. This means *not* complaining loudly about strange (to you) customs, bragging that they make it/cook it/do it better back home, raising your voice a decibel to make some dumb foreigner understand a simple question in plain English, or wearing your ignorance of the land and people you are visiting like a badge.

If a place is worth visiting, then it's surely worth reading about before you go. Just a little bit of homework will dispel much of the awkwardness that comes from not knowing how to cope in a foreign clime, and it's certain to make your trip more rewarding and enjoyable to boot. A phrase book, a good guide book, and an open, appreciative attitude are all you need to set you apart—far apart—from J. J. Blowhard of Topeka, Kansas, who never understands why he can't get two eggs over easy with soft bacon and white toast for breakfast in Paris, France. *Vive la différence!*

MARRIAGE

Saying that it's better to marry than to burn at the stake isn't saying much. What about: It's better to marry than to go dateless on Friday night? Not to mention: It's better to marry than to lie in bed with the flu with nobody to fluff your pillows, make your tea, and read you the box scores? Makes you want to run right out, find Ms. Right, and tie the knot.

There is no question, though, that marriage is serious stuff, not to be entered into lightly, even if it does mean fluffy pillows. Marriage is like cohabitation only more so—no hedging of bets this time. The name of the game is sharing, and it's supposed to last forever.

So congratulations! You're a family unit! Now when you say you're going home for Thanksgiving or Christmas, you have every right to be referring to *your* place, not Mom and Dad's. And since the honeymoon is over, we thought we'd offer a little marital advice.

NAMES

You don't have to change yours, so why should she change hers? Well, it's not always quite that simple. Like a wedding ring for the groom (see below), the name change for the bride is often the subject of hot debate, with some pretty dubious reasoning attached ("If you really loved me, you'd want to change your name to mine . . .").

Everyone knows that a woman has the right to keep her name (and that it probably makes sense for a woman not to change names once she's got her career going), but a lot of men can't help but get their feelings hurt. If you're one of them, by all means tell her how you feel, but honor her decision without whining.

MONEY

As we said, one of the most important aspects of marriage is sharing, and we're not just talking about space in the medicine cabinet. We mean money, too. Many couples regard joint accounts with a jaundiced eye—they prefer separate checking accounts and splitting expenses—but no matter how you handle it, you'll have to get over the practical and psychological hurdles of sharing the wealth. The more you talk about it—honestly and quietly if you can manage it—the better off you'll be.

Figure out what kind of checking system makes sense. Decide who will carry which credit cards and whether you should be co-signators. (If women are smart, they'll keep all the credit cards they had before marrying. Once you start telling department stores about your personal life, nothing good can happen.)

Make a deal that neither of you will spend more than a given amount—$100, $500, whatever—without checking with the other first, and that you'll discuss all major purchases before hitting the stores. You'll be amazed at how many financial disagreements can be prevented this way.

When April 15 rolls around, you'll have to do some more sharing—this time with the IRS. Romance and/or protocol have nothing whatsoever to do with the decision of whether to file separately or jointly. This is when Cupid takes a back seat to your accountant.

RINGS

Since time immemorial, men have resisted wearing wedding rings, and women have been unhappy about it. This unhappiness can be manifested by anything from mild hurt to wild anger, and like the question of name-changing (see above), it can engender some pretty illogical dialogue ("If you really loved me, you'd want to wear a ring so that people would know we're married . . .").

Wearing a ring is less of an imposition than changing a name, but it's still *your* decision. While it behooves a guy to take his wife's wishes and feelings into account, he does get to choose his own jewelry.

TOGETHERNESS

People magazine articles and *Lifestyles of the Rich and Famous* segments notwithstanding, we're not big believers in bi-coastal marriages, frequent separate vacations, or even a whole lot of separate socializing for married couples. There's no law that says that you and the missus have to be joined at the hip—and they do say that absence makes the heart grown fonder—but presumably you got married so that you could spend some time together.

When you're invited to a party, assume that your wife is welcome—and expected. Check with her before accepting any invitation. (She doesn't have to go, but she does have to be told about it.) As hard as it may be to accept, your days of going stag or being the extra man at a dinner party are over. Period.

IN-LAWS

You don't have to love and cherish her parents and promise to spend all holidays with them, but even if it's sheer torture you have to be cordial and polite and let them have a look at their daughter and her husband once in a while. And the same goes for her—even if she can't stand your folks, she has to make an effort. You can make separate visits to your respective homesteads occasionally, but every once in a while you must show the flag together. Otherwise they'll start to worry.

By the way, calling her parents Mom and Dad is a little silly even if you're wild about them (it's possible). Unless that comes very naturally to you, we suggest that you opt for using their first names.

ARGUING

Three observations:

1. All arguments are about sex, money, housework, and in-laws.

2. A marital spat should never take place in public.
3. You really *shouldn't* go to bed mad.

(See also COHABITATION, MONEY, CREDIT CARDS, WEDDING, and DIVORCE.)

MONEY

John and Paul were right: Money can't buy you love. But it can buy other things (see AUTOMOBILES), it does make the world go 'round, and it matters more to most people than sex. At least that's what Alfred Kinsey suspected when he started asking people about their sex lives 40 years ago. They talked freely about what took place in their bedrooms, but they clammed up about how much money they earned.

There are three good rules to live by when it comes to money: (1) Don't flaunt it; (2) Don't get too serious about it as a life goal; and (3) Be generous. If you go through life paying just a little more than your share, you'll never regret it, even though it means dividing the lunch tab by four when all you had was the chicken salad on whole wheat.

Now, here are the answers to some of your other money questions:

How should I behave if I have more money than my friends do? Like the cat who swallowed the canary. And you should also devise strategies for spending more on your friends than they can afford to spend on you without making them feel awkward and embarrassed. This will involve stating explicitly that "I want you to be my guests tonight" when suggesting a restaurant that's more expensive than their norm. It can mean telling a white lie about precisely how you came to get four 50-yard-line seats for the big game that's been sold out for months. And it certainly means receiving as well as giving—that is, not grabbing every tab automatically (see rule one: Don't flaunt it), but letting your friends treat you from time to time. It's called reciprocity, and it helps keep friendship on an even keel even though bank accounts aren't.

What if I have less money than my friends do? You're not likely to start sticking up convenience stores, so you might as well practice not getting bent out of shape about anything extraneous that really shouldn't affect your friendships, like money. There is no necessary connection, after all, between money and intelligence, ethics, goodness, or badness. And there are too many ways to reciprocate that don't involve money (or much of it) for you to fret about not being able to afford champagne for everybody.

Should I ever borrow money from friends? Only if they own a bank. The old adage "Neither a borrower nor a lender be" is particularly true when it comes to friends. There's nothing more likely to break up a friendship than money loaned, unless it's a wife swapped.

Is it ever okay to give money as a gift? Only if the recipient is under 21, in which case it's strongly preferred.

Is money the root of all evil? No, something else is.

MOTHER'S DAY

M is for the many times you forgot to send a card or a present, you rat, you! And after she carried you for nine months! As long as flowers and candy and balloons can be sent through the mail on the same day you order them, there's really no excuse for missing this one. If you'd care to give it just a little more thought, you can't go wrong with a nice card and perfume, jewelry, a scarf, a book, or a picture of you, her favorite son. If you're only going to call, at least call early in the day and put her out of her misery.

MOVIES

Let's face it—there's no way that watching movies at home on a VCR will ever take the place of the real thing. For one thing, at home they won't let you throw your trash on the floor. No, we're going to be going out to the movies for a long time. So let's take a moment to set some ground rules for movie theater behavior.

It goes without saying that you don't talk, kick the chair in front of you, or eat Moo Goo Gai Pan in a movie theater. But what's to be done about people who do?

First of all, accept the fact that there are people in the world who don't care if their talking or kicking or eating or smoking is bothering you. Maybe they need a lot of understanding and a couple of years in therapy, but that's not the point. The point is that after you've said, "Quiet, please," and "Will you stop kicking my chair, please?" you've pretty much said it all. Don't holler, threaten, or otherwise lose your temper. A person who would kick your chair is perfectly capable of punching your lights out or even setting fire to the theater. Change seats. If there's no place in the theater where you can enjoy the movie in peace, ask for your money back.

NEW YEAR'S EVE

New Year's Eve is the strangest of all holidays—even when you have fun, you end up being at least mildly depressed. No matter what your age or marital status, you basically can't win for losing: If you decide to go to a party, you end up wishing you'd had dinner with the lady of your choice or perhaps a few close friends. If you keep the festivities small, you wind up thinking you're a complete dullard with no friends. And there's no point in pretending that it's just another day. You can try it, of course, but around about midnight you'll start hankering for Guy Lombardo and a paper hat and someone special to kiss.

The best way to get around the whole problem is tradition—find something you like to do (and preferably someone you like to do it with) and then do it every year. This can be as simple as pizza and an all-night poker game with five college buddies or Chinese food and *The Godfather* on your VCR at home, or something as elaborate as dinner and dancing at the most expensive hotel in town, or a long weekend at the ski resort of your choice. The more predictable you can make it, the better. That way you don't have to choose from the same unsatisfying options every year.

This way can lie heartbreak, of course. Friends move away, dancing partners change, and some people don't like poker or *The Godfather*. That's when it's time to think up a new tradition.

Anyway, cheer up! It could be worse. You could be one of those poor souls whose birthday is December 31.

NO (HOW TO SAY IT)

You've been there before.

At a cocktail party, standing with a warm drink in your hand, penned into a corner by your host's cousin, who with nasal voice and shrimpy breath spends thirteen minutes on a detailed exegesis of a new book about satan worship. Or at a friend's home for Sunday brunch, the hidden agenda of which is to fix you up with Ms. Right, only she's all wrong. Or at a noisy, crowded restaurant, where you discover over appetizers that neither you nor your companion has anything to say to the other, you both know it, and dessert is still at least an hour and eighty-five dollars away.

What's at issue here is pretty basic: how to get control of your own life and stop playing the leading man in social nightmares that can usually be avoided simply by knowing how to say "No."

Yes, it's not all that easy. Acquaintances intrude on time intended for friends. Social and business lives overlap. Deciding how to allocate energy and commitment takes on the proportions of resource distribution in a marginal economy: too much demand, not enough supply.

It's also true that if you're currently unattached, not too happy with the fact, and sitting at home watching a *Taxi* rerun, a call asking you to fill the single man's chair at a dinner party two weeks from Tuesday is going to sound mighty swell, no matter that it comes from a matched set of bores. And if you're feeling particularly insecure, as any normal person does from time to time, declining that social engagement is going to seem like a high-risk proposition ("What if no one ever invites me to anything ever again, as long as I live?").

But saying no is an important skill you should master and use, precisely because it enables you to free up blocks of time for those things—family, relationships, personal interests, professional growth, putting topspin on your backhand—that matter most.

The first thing you have to do is rid yourself of guilt. Declining an invitation isn't likely to make your would-be hosts change their names and move out of town in shame. Friends will survive your absence. So will your friendships.

Declining an invitation for a specific date or event shouldn't present a problem. "I'm sorry, I have other plans" works nicely and is unassailable. No need to go beyond that. "I'll have to check my calendar and get back to you" is okay too, but be sure to do so within twenty-four hours at the most. Any longer and you'll look like a free agent holding out for a better offer.

"You pick the date" and "If Tuesday's no good, any day the following week" from would-be hosts are tougher to parry, but "I'm going to be traveling a lot in the next few weeks, so I'm really not able to make any plans right now" will put things off for a while. Two doses of this, administered graciously, should do the trick.

Remember the TV ad a few years ago in which a gorgeous woman calls a man to ask if she can drop by? The last ten seconds of the half-minute drama establish that she already knows the guy passingly well, and the reason for the visit is to bring him a bottle of expensive booze as a gift. Never mind that she's too perfect to have ever even contemplated rejection, much less experienced it. The vignette still reflects a relatively new development in relations between the sexes: Woman calls Man.

Most men are so accustomed to doing the asking, and particularly to the anxiety associated with anticipating the answer, that we should be sensitive to the nuances of saying no. Should be but aren't. So the next time you're on the receiving end of an invitation for a date from a woman, be sure to give yourself a quick reality check.

If the chemistry's dead wrong, and you knew it the minute you met at that dreadful cocktail party—if, say, she likes early John Denver and late Bob Dylan and her favorite novelist is James Fenimore Cooper—don't be so dazzled by the newness of a woman doing the asking that your lips say yes while your head whispers no. Just remember the times when you asked someone out, there was a pause, and then a yes that really meant (or sounded like it meant), "I am stunned that you would even dream of asking, but I'm not doing anything next Tuesday and I haven't been to Lutèce in a while." Saying yes that way is more cruel than the bluntest no.

Sometimes the signals won't be clear. She may have baseball tickets to the company box, she knows you're a fan, and sees you as a potential client. Period. On the other hand, maybe the first two statements are true, but romantic interest has pinch-hit for the third. It makes a difference. And if the invitation is for lunch, ask yourself if she has business or pleasure in mind. Figure wrong on this and you'll end up hoping for food poisoning to end your agony. Consider: The key to understanding her intentions may be to understand yours first.

As with invitations from other sectors, saying no when a woman calls is easy if a specified date is involved. Just don't sound too disappointed at not being free ("Gosh darn, gee whiz, I'd really like to, but I've had these plans forever"), lest you elicit an unwanted counterproposal for another evening. If the invitation is a general one ("Would you like to have dinner sometime?"), you can ease into a no with small talk (one friend deftly deflects suitors by casually mentioning enough allergies and eccentricities that the poor caller ends up feeling relieved at being rejected), followed by vague commitments ("Things are particularly hectic at work right now"), and ending with a distancing alternative ("Maybe next month").

This approach may not work, of course. She may not take this sort of no for an answer. So you must be prepared, if pressed, to say, "I just don't think it makes sense for the two of us to see each other." Don't feel compelled to go into detail. Honesty may be the best policy, but full disclosure frequently isn't. Save your "painful but true" observations for relationships that have gone sour and call for termination with causes spelled out.

Sometimes you'll find yourself wanting to say, "No, not now." This means that the spirit is willing but the flesh has other plans. Don't be coy, but do make it clear that you're flattered, and that seeing her would be great under other circumstances. Do not, however, feel obligated to spell them out if they muddy the water ("I don't want to get involved with anyone until the divorce papers have been signed" isn't very romantic). Next time, of course, it's your nickel.

No (How to Take It Like a Man)

Easy. Just pretend it doesn't matter at all, no matter how much it does.

PARENTS

Some psychiatrists say that the distance you put between yourself and your parents when you were a teenager was a necessary part of growing up. Maybe so. But sometimes it seems that the distance we put between ourselves and our parents now is a measure (not the only one by any means, but a biggie) of how grown up we really are. Even certified public accountants and brain surgeons are kids when they go home to see Mom and Dad.

Of course, the generation gap is always with us, and it's a rare parent-child relationship indeed that is without tension. More power to you if you can relax and be yourself when you are with your parents, but if avoiding World War III during an occasional visit is more your speed, consider the following:

• They're your parents, after all, and chances are you see them only a couple times a year. Why start a huge fight about politics or religion or your marital status or your job or your taste in clothes or the designated hitter rule when tomorrow you'll be back home? Bite your tongue.

• Don't expect your folks to understand exactly what you do for a living. We're not sure why, but most parents just can't manage this. If you like talking shop, ask your folks for advice about a business problem.

• Always ask your mother to cook your favorite dish, the one you remember so fondly from childhood. If there is no such dish, make one up. And while you're at it, ask your dad for one of his great Harvey Wallbangers.

• Think about it long and hard before taking a woman home to meet the folks. They're bound to think that the visit is a prelude to the wedding rehearsal dinner, and you can hardly blame them. So don't introduce just everyone to Mom and Dad. On the other hand, it's only fair that Ms. Right and your parents should at least get a look at one another before the grandchildren arrive. When the meeting day does come, make it as casual as possible and choose neutral territory, by which we mean as far from your baby pictures as you can manage. Dinner at a nice informal restaurant should do nicely. Tact is the order of the day.

• Ever since the good old days when you had to remind your folks about your allowance, money has probably played a significant part in your family affairs. Now that you're getting a regular paycheck and stopped shaking cards and letters from the folks to see if a greenback falls out, that part is probably smaller, but it may not have disappeared entirely. As far as protocol is concerned, if your folks want to give you a few bucks, you should probably take them. There's no point in arguing about it, and besides, it's a lot better than having them cut your meat for you.

• Have children of your own right away. Your parents won't ever want to talk to you again except to offer to baby-sit while you and your wife take that trip to Antarctica you've always dreamed about.

(See also MOTHER'S DAY, FATHER'S DAY, and CHILDREN.)

POKER

Unquestionably the world's greatest indoor sport, poker always has been, and always will be, a man's game. A lot of bona fide men don't play, of course, and a lot of women play a whole lot better than a lot of men want to believe, but poker is quintessentially masculine. Virtually every American male over the age of 21 will, at some point, be asked to play cards with the guys some Wednesday night. A substantial majority will say yes, at least once. Many will go on to do it on a fairly regular basis. And some will embrace poker as one of the essential ingredients of a rich, full life.

Here are some things to think about if you fit into any of the above categories. Some have to do with your mental approach, some with the etiquette of poker. All are discrete elements of a grander whole. None deal directly with the abiding lure and extraordinary lore of the game, which are worthy of a lifetime's dedication. But each helps clear your mind so you can focus all your psychic energy on not shouting "Hot damn!" when you draw that third ace.

The play's the thing. Keep the chatter down. You're sitting around the table to play poker, not to rehash the week's triumphs and tragedies on other fronts. And just because you've spent some mighty fine hours in other locales with one or more of the guys at the table debating the relative strength of the Dodgers and the Yankees does not give you *carte blanche* to bring up batting averages between deals. The game should be social—you're there to have fun with friends—but poker comes first, at least tonight.

Money matters. Never play for stakes that are too high or too low. If five guys are comfortable with a win-lose swing of $150 per session, but a sixth really can't afford to lose more than $50 without it hurting something other than his self-esteem, get a new sixth. That may sound harsh, but putting a friend in a position where he must routinely risk more than he can afford to lose is not a friendly act. On the other hand, poker is nothing without tension, bluff, and hunch, and dropping the stakes so low that the other players lose interest will surely kill the game. It's a tough call, but if you want to have a good poker game, you have to build it with people for whom betting a kings-over boat to the hilt and losing a $100 pot to four threes has approximately the same financial consequences. It should sting, but it shouldn't keep anyone's little sister from having the operation she needs so she'll be able to walk like all the other girls.

Last call. Poker is timeless, but you have to sleep. What to do? Agree on a quitting time before the first hand is dealt. If you're sitting in as a substitute and no one else says anything about time, it's perfectly okay to announce as you sit down that you have to leave at 1:00 a.m. (It's even okay to add "or a hundred dollars down, whichever comes first.") If you're a regular, any major departure from your game's norm—such as being able to play only until 10:00 p.m., when the game usually ends at midnight—should be duly reported to everyone before the night of the game so the others can decide whether to get a replacement for you. Don't feel hurt if they do—removing one-sixth of a table two-thirds of the way into the game will drastically alter inner tempos and silent melodies.

Playing the hand that's dealt you. Every poker game develops its own special personality. Loose, easy, an excuse to get together. Or tight, intense, the game's the thing. Between those points is a broad spectrum of nuances and shadings. Normally, you can tell after one round of deals in an established game whether it's for you. Chances are it won't be, since it evolved to this point with someone else in the chair you're now sitting in. You can have fun, but never come to an established game expecting to feel comfortable instantly, and don't believe for a moment that you'll be able to remake it to match your notion of what an ideal poker game ought to be. Might as well try to hijack a ship of fools.

A time to fish, a time to cut bait. Till death do us part isn't any more binding in poker than it is in marriage, so be prepared to walk away from a game if it goes sour. Don't worry, you'll be able to spot the signs. Ed saying, "Let-me-see, let-me-see, let-me-see," to himself *sotto voce* every time he spreads his hand or takes a peek at his hole cards . . . Ben, who is right-handed, dealing left-handed, very slowly . . . Jerry, the host, who owns a state-of-the-art answering machine, stopping play every time the phone rings to take the call . . . Tom/Dick/Harry always, *always* having to be reminded that it's his turn to bet, to deal, to shuffle, to "Ante up, goddammit!"

By the time you become fully, consciously aware of all these irritants—which have been growing like fungi since the game was young and fresh, after all—it's too late to do a darned thing about them. Frank talk with the offenders will only add insult (to them) or injury (to you). Cut your losses and walk.

One last thing. If you sit down at a poker table and a smartly dressed fellow with a pencil-thin mustache bets you $100 that he can make the king of diamonds jump out of the deck and squirt vinegar in your ear, don't call the bet.

PUNCTUALITY

In the course of human history, punctuality is a fairly recent value. From the Middle Ages through the Napoleonic Era, people in the Western World depended on church bells to tell them it was time for morning, midday, or evening religious services. Not until the 19th century, when railroad timetables came into being, was it necessary for large numbers of people to know the exact time. Need begat invention, and the development and manufacture of reliable personal timepieces—the pocket watches carried by our great-grandfathers—made it possible for gentlemen in the Industrial Age to be on time. In our decade, of course, wristwatches are so readily available that one fashion fad involves wearing three, four, or more at the same time. Talk about *reductio ad absurdam:* Nowadays it's virtually impossible *not* to know what time it is.

Enough history. What about the etiquette of time and punctuality? Whether you are on time may be a matter of easily ascertainable fact, but whether that is also the *right* time to arrive or depart is a matter of social convention.

Dinner at eight. Unless your hosts are calling out for pizza, the time of a dinner invitation is not something to be trifled with. Eight o'clock means 8:00 to 8:15, period. After that, your hosts' kitchen schedule is thrown off. They'll smile, but they'll hate you for it.

The only thing worse than arriving late for a dinner party is arriving early. Show up at 7:45 and you're apt to find your hosts half-dressed and dashing around the kitchen trying to compress an hour's preparations into 15 minutes. They're praying all their guests still believe in arriving fashionably late and here you are, ready for a cocktail.

Cocktails, 6:00 to 8:00. If your hosts are close friends, get there promptly at 6:00. Nobody likes to be first, and there's nothing deadlier than the first half hour of a cocktail party. But it's a tough time for hosts. Even the steeliest of souls may wonder,

"Is anybody going to show?" So get there on time, show the flag, and your friends will rest easier.

The less acquainted you are with the people giving the affair, the less important it is when you arrive—up to a point. And that point, for an invitation that specifies 6:00 to 8:00, is 7:15. When people stipulate a time frame for a party, you should always consider the last half hour as a time for leave-taking, not a time for showing up, so arriving 7:15 gives you a quarter hour for saying hello before you can politely say goodbye.

Get me to the church on time. And to the theater, the movies, the ballgame, or any other event that starts promptly at an appointed hour. There is no exemplar of rudeness more despicable than the movie latecomer who blocks your view of the credits and tromps your feet as he stumbles toward the vacant seats in the middle of the row seconds after the rest of the house has finally stopped yapping. Odds are he will be the one in every movie theater who feels compelled to interpret the more subtle scenes for his companion in a loud stage whisper. Odds are better that he will miss the point. Don't be him.

Fashionably late. Forget it. There's no such thing.

RESTAURANTS

Some fancy restaurants have all the charm and appeal of a minefield. Unfamiliar cutlery, intimidating wine lists, arrogant wine stewards, an unwritten but rigid dress code, haughty waiters, and menus written in foreign languages are just a half dozen of the obstacles seemingly designed to ruin your evening. The number of digits in the check is another.

Dealing with the last is between you and your state lottery, but there are steps you can take to put yourself in control of the rest.

Ordering for her. In olden days a lady seated in a restaurant with a gentleman was forbidden by prevailing standards of etiquette to speak to waiters, presumably because direct contact could be considered forward. Maybe our ancestors feared that "I'll have the veal" from a lady's lips carried the subliminal message "My place or yours?" to a waiter's ears. Or maybe they thought a gender that was genetically unsuited to offering toasts or taking charge of business meetings couldn't be expected to deal with even the simplest of public announcements. Whatever the reasoning, the prohibition meant that a lady's dining companion had to memorize her menu choices—no mean task if the menu was in French or she was a big eater—and pass on this information to the waiter without stumbling over a sauce or confusing a cooking instruction.

Younger waiters these days are generally too preoccupied with their acting careers to ask if you're ready to order. And after they've told you their name and recited the house specials, they stand poised to accept your applause, not your choice of entrées. But relics of the *ancien régime* abound, particularly in the smarter places, the kind where a small bowl of soup costs seven dollars. What should you do if one of these haughty veterans of the old school of waitering by intimidation marches up to the table, looks you dead in the eye, and says, "Are you ready to order, sir?"

Simple. Unless you suspect the kitchen is running short of the surf 'n' turf you've been thinking about since midafternoon, you turn to your female companion and ask, "Have you decided?" This signals the waiter that it's okay to address the woman directly—"Roquefort or creamy garlic?"—without asking your permission or prompting a fainting spell. You are thus spared the trouble of having to play United Nations' interpreter, and she gets to behave like a grown-up.

And—who knows—letting a woman speak for herself in a restaurant may even cause the newly liberated waiter, hitherto oblivious to the existence of female patrons independent enough to order their own food, to place the check equidistant between you and your dining partner when the meal has been completed. Dare to dream.

Bad service. A restaurant is more than food, and a waiter is more than someone who brings it to you. Arrogance, indifference, rudeness, and incompetence—though encountered in roadside diner and four-star beanery alike, and sometimes perversely perceived in the latter as a symptom of excellence—should not be tolerated.

After all, it's the waiter's job to help you over the rough spots on a strange menu, gently nudge you toward a sensible choice of wines, and pretend that you're a splendid fellow to boot. No discordant notes, thank you. You're perfectly capable of screwing up an evening without any help from strangers.

If you are treated badly, complain. Easier said than done if you've just moved up a notch on the fancy level, you're the youngest person in the joint, and the waiter has just given you one of those looks usually reserved for younger brothers who've just done something uncool. But complain you must, or the lout will fork and twist you like a strand of spaghetti.

But not to the waiter. Go over his head to the captain, the maître d'hôtel, the manager, the owner, the varlet's boss, whatever the title. State your case quietly and ask—also quietly—to be assigned a new waiter or moved to a different table. Chances are he won't, but if it's a class place he will—quietly—jerk a knot in the offender and get him on the right track.

Do this in midmeal only if the service has been atrocious. Save it till afterward if it's been merely bad. You can tell from the response whether the person in charge appreciates the value of addressing a customer's legitimate complaints. If not, this isn't the sort of place you'll be coming back to anyway. If you do get a sympathetic hearing, make a point of coming back soon.

Whatever you do, don't leave the restaurant without registering your gripe, even if the place is a trendy hotspot perfectly capable of getting away for months, maybe longer, with doling out equal measures of lousy food and worse service—and without your patronage, thank you. So what if nothing you could possibly say is likely to change things? Saying your piece anyway—the right way, to the right person—will make you feel better and salvage something of the evening. The good part.

Bad food. A tougher call than bad service because food is . . . well, a matter of taste. We're not talking here about meat ordered rare but delivered well-done, or anything lukewarm that should be hot. Such matters are taken up with the waiter and corrected promptly (in the best of all possible worlds).

But what if you're not sure how an unfamiliar dish is supposed to taste? Most of us weren't brought up on curried snails, and who are we to say we think there's a tad too much cardamom in them? Sulking will turn your mood sour, and just saying it's lousy doesn't ameliorate the problem. Instead, ask the waiter to return the dish to the chef for tasting. This is a class move, because it implies you trust everyone to behave honorably. People respect that and are more likely to take the high road if they think you expect it of them. The best that can happen is that the chef will agree with you, and you'll get to try something else, while winning points all around for good taste and good manners. The worst is that you can learn once and for all that you really don't like curried snails, no matter how well they're prepared, thus saving you from future disappointment.

Of course, if everyone at your table gets bad food, it can mean only one thing: a bad restaurant. Mark it down to experience, agree to have dessert somewhere else, and suggest to the owner-manager as you leave that he should consider another line of work.

Wine. There's more nonsense written about wine than about anything else in the world, with the possible exception of art, and just as much posturing about it by people who have nothing better to show off about.

If all you know about wine is red with meat and white with fish, go with the house wine until you teach yourself something more. You can also ask the waiter or the wine steward for advice, but be prepared to ignore it if the only recommendations are the three highest-priced bottles on the list. There's no point in risking major bucks when you have no basis for evaluating the return on your investment. Learning about wine by drinking it frequently is the best way, and virtually guaranteed to enhance your appreciation of one of life's most pleasant experiences. But restaurant prices make for high tuition, so do your studying at home—at least until you have a grasp of the basics. (See also WINE.)

When you order wine in a restaurant, ask for the wine list and then find out what everyone at the table is planning to eat. With luck everyone will be having fish and chicken (white) or chicken and meat (red). If it doesn't work out that way, don't start shredding menus and demanding pitchers of beer. Just look for half bottles on the list or take a deep breath and order a full bottle of each. Take as long as you like over the wine list, ignoring pushy waiters and others overeager to help. It's no shame to ask for advice if you can't make up your mind. In good restaurants the wine steward may well know what he is talking about. When the wine arrives, the waiter or wine steward will pour a bit into your glass. Swirl it and inhale the bouquet, and sip. Then, if all's well, signal your approval. And that's that. If the wine tastes "off," say so, and ask for another choice. You might also ask the steward for corroboration.

But whatever you do, however much you learn about wine, do not turn the drinking of it into an elaborate ceremony. It's better simple.

The tip. Fifteen percent for adequate service (see more under TIPPING), and that may be as little as remembering who gets the fries in a burger joint. But you'll certainly expect more from a waiter wherever there's more than one fork by your plate. Up to 20 percent for outstanding service (such as recommending a great dish, warning you away from an overpriced wine, and being present but not omnipresent, informed but not officious, cordial but not chummy). A captain or maìtre d'hôtel who explains things and helps you orchestrate the meal gets 5 percent, a wine steward 5 percent of the price of the wine.

More means that you're from out of town or that this is a very, very special evening and everyone has pulled out the stops. Less means that you're from out or town or that the service has been subpar (in which case you should reinforce the tip's message by alerting someone in the restaurant's hierarchy to the problem). Don't make the mistake of undertipping as a form of punishment just because the food is bad. The waiter didn't cook the swill, and he didn't order it, so he shouldn't be punished just for bringing it.

ROOMMATE

I f you have a roommate, you can probably write your own book on the subject, so here are a few pointers for those just embarking on that wonderful experience. Of course, you have your own room. Of course, you have either your own bathroom or a time worked out when it may as well be yours. Of course, you've long since worked out how you and your roommate will deal with utilities and shop for, pay for, cook, and eat the food in the apartment. You've agreed to split the cost of a weekly cleaning woman, and you've graduated from the *Animal House* approach to entertaining a visitor of the opposite sex. Why, then, aren't you happy? Because you haven't discovered the secret to the perfect roommate relationship: your very own phone, with its own number and its own answering machine (see ANSWERING MACHINES).

Of course there's more to harmony between roommates than that, but virtually everything else can be dealt with or gotten around by the exercise of common sense and common courtesy. Let him know if you're having company (of any sort) and ask him to do the same. Establish ground rules about where such company will be entertained, and, if you're both very sociable indeed, how often each of you will put up with it. Don't take advantage of your roommate and don't let him take advantage of you.

If you're seeing a woman who has a roommate, take all your cues from her when you're at her place. If you have an apartment all to yourself, you'll probably feel most comfortable seeing her at your home, but there may be times when you'll want to stop in at her place, if only for a short visit. If you end up spending a lot of time at her apartment, make a contribution that can be enjoyed by her roommate as well: Replenish the liquor cabinet, buy a plant for the living room, order some firewood, or pay to have the paper delivered.

In these anything-can-happen, particularly-with-rents-so-high Eighties, you may end up sharing your apartment with a woman.

In general, coed living has its advantages (the apartment usually looks and smells better) and its disadvantages (unspeakable things in the bathroom), but open discussions and well thought-out ground rules will almost always make for harmonious life. Be sure to clear the air about sleep-over dates and use of the bathroom.

RSVP

By our highly unscientific estimates, we figure that about half the people who receive an invitation with the initials RSVP at the bottom will ignore them. We're not sure why. Maybe they're rude, inconsiderate dolts. Maybe they don't understand French abbreviations.

If it's the first reason, only prayer will help, but we can give you a hand with the second. RSVP stands for *répondez s'il vous plâit,* and that's a very nice, old-fashioned way of saying *please respond.* So please do.

The nicest, classiest way to respond to a written invitation is to write a nice note, but even Emily Post herself would say that it's acceptable to make a phone call, particularly since that's what most people without live-in secretarial help do anyway. It's common these days for the telephone number for RSVPs to appear on the invitation. If it does, feel free to use it. When you do call (promptly, please), do it with style—resist the impulse to use RSVP as a verb. Don't say, "I'm calling to RSVP." Say, "I'm calling to accept with pleasure your invitation to get down and boogie on Saturday next."

And speaking of things not to do, there are few things in life more tacky than those little response cards ("Check one: Yes, I will attend. No, I will not be able to attend.") that sometimes accompany formal invitations. The folks who send them undoubtedly mean well—they probably think that those coupons save their friends a gang of trouble—but reducing a nice social function to a mail-order transaction is not our idea of style. If you're doing the inviting, let the nice people write their own notes. After all, what else are they going to use their stationery for?

(See also COCKTAIL PARTIES, DINNER PARTY, INVITATIONS, and STATIONERY.)

SETTING A TABLE

Unless you're a ranking diplomat or a social snob devising tests to identify interlopers, the cardinal rule for setting a table is, Keep It Simple. The goal is to create an environment that's pleasing rather than demanding, and to make your guests feel comfortable rather than intimidated. On Thanksgiving Day it's fine to trot out every piece of silverware and fine china you own, not to mention those terrific antique place-card holders Uncle Pete gave you. But the rest of the year, less is usually more.

Napkins. The best case that can be made for polyester blends is that they let you use cloth napkins at every meal with little hassle or expense. Linen napkins are great, but they cost about 75 cents apiece to have cleaned. Paper napkins are okay for pizza and picnics, and the cocktail size are good for cocktails.

Flatware. Sterling silver is swell, but a handsome set of stainless steel is more versatile for life on the go.

Dinnerware. The same is true for bone china and simple stoneware. Great if you have it, but you can still set a splendid table if you don't.

Candles. Always add ambiance, but elegant candleholders should be held back for special occasions and *très intime* dinners for two (so long as it isn't the first date). Easy to go overboard here, so use restraint, and make sure your candles don't remind anyone of Liberace.

Tablecloths. Freshly ironed linen is grand, and a must for the most formal dinner parties. But the practical and good-looking blends available today are another good reason for saluting breeders of polyester. (Mind you, we're talking at least 40-percent natural fabric content; all-polyester causes indigestion.)

Wineglasses. Wine tradition says you are supposed to have differently shaped glasses for red and white wine, but you can get by nicely with an all-purpose stemmed glass so long as it is the right one—large (10 to 14 ounces capacity, even though you never pour more than 6) and tulip-shaped or rounded (make sure the opening is slightly smaller in circumference than the middle).

Flowers. Always welcome, except for lilies and marigolds.

Layout. Silver or stainless steel is placed in the order of its use, with the implements to be used first farthest from the plate. (The one exception is a seafood fork, used for a first course of, say, mussels or shrimp; this will appear to the extreme right, beyond the spoons.) Thus, if you're serving soup, a main course, a salad course, and dessert, you would set the table as follows. Starting from the left of the plate: folded napkin, dinner fork, salad fork. And to the right of the plate: dinner knife (blade turned inward), soup spoon, teaspoon. Above, left: bread and butter plate, with butter knife laid on it. Above, right: wineglass(es), with first to be used on the right if you use more than one, and water goblet, if used, on the right. Above, center: dessert fork or spoon with handle on right. (You may instead bring on dessert implements at the time dessert is served.)

This layout, of course, is for a full-court, no-holds-barred, hit-them-with-your-best-shot dinner for six or more. It would look kind of dopey for a couple of friends who dropped over for pasta and a salad. But, hey, life isn't a beer commercial. Unfortunately.

SHOPPING

What on earth, you might well ask, is an entry on Shopping doing in a guide to modern manners? Do I have to be told not to shove to the front of a cash register line the week before Christmas, even if TIME IS RUNNING OUT? Of course not, any more than you have to be reminded that certain stores in some towns—Bloomingdale's in New York, for example—have a local reputation as hot spots for meeting people of the opposite sex.

The reason for having an entry on Shopping is to make the point that you can't be adept at giving gifts (see GIFTS) unless you know what's out there on the market. And the time to learn is not the day the gift is to be presented.

So think of shopping as research, not as buying. Skip lunch someday and spend an hour browsing through a store or two to see what's available. Don't speak to anyone except for the necessary "No, thank you's" to queries from salespeople, and above all, don't buy anything—not a single thing.

Time wasted/opportunities missed? Not on your life. It's money saved and peace of mind won the next time the occasion for a gift pops up on your calendar.

SMOKING

Slowly but surely, the world as we once knew it is being divided into two opposing camps—people who smoke (aka Smokers) and people who don't (Nonsmokers). Okay, maybe this division doesn't carry with it the threat of thermonuclear war, but it is increasingly the cause of harsh words and hurt feelings. What this world does not need right now is another issue to tear people apart and set them at each other's throats, so let's sit and reason together, with the common goal of peaceful coexistence.

If you don't smoke, don't go out of your way to be mean to people who do. Look at it this way: Most people who smoke feel guilty and terrible about it, they're probably trying their darnedest to stop, and negative pressure from you will only make matters worse. You have specific legal rights, to be sure, along with legitimate expectations of fair consideration from others. You have an absolutely effective alternative—not hanging out with smokers. And you also have time, social pressure, growing public awareness, even the government (with one big exception: federal price support for tobacco) on your side.

If you *do* smoke, remember that it's a hostile world out there, and you'd be wise to practice Defensive Smoking. Among other things, this means that you should:

- Ask before lighting up around other people;
- Be prepared to take "No, I'd prefer it if you didn't" for an answer (and take it graciously);
- Be particularly careful about confined spaces;
- Obey No Smoking signs without bursting into tears or ripping them off the wall;
- Stay on the alert to body language and other subtle tipoffs that a Nonsmoking zealot is nearby and waiting to pounce (it is a fact of life that the people who give you a hard time for smoking will inevitably do so in a loud voice);
- Be prepared to concede all constitutional debates with Non-

smokers, no matter how much you believe that lighting up is an inalienable right;

• Come to grips with the reality that "Smoking Can Be—make that, *Is*—Hazardous to Your Social Health."

As for you Nonsmokers, go ahead and be vigilant about your right to breathe clean air. But be understanding as well: A lot of your friends want to stop every bit as much as you want them to. Practice politeness ("Excuse me, this is a nonsmoking area" or "Please, do you mind not smoking?") rather than confrontation ("Hey, put it out! Can't you read the sign?" or "Get rid of the cigarette, buster, or I'll punch your lights out!"). And—here's a free civics lesson—be careful about asking the government to pass laws telling people what they can and can't do, particularly in an area where they've always done as they damned well please.

SPORTSMANSHIP

The word amateur is commonly used in our culture to describe a job done poorly, as in "He played like a rank amateur" or "It was an amateurish production." It's become a term of denigration, and that's a pity, because the original meaning of the word had nothing to do with *how* someone did something, but with *why* he did it. "Amateur" derives from the Latin *amare,* "to love," and refers to someone who does something simply for the love of doing it.

In sports the amateur used to be an athlete whose love of playing and competing was fulfillment enough, whose motive for performing to the best of his ability had nothing to do with money or any other reward save love of the sport. This is important to keep in mind, because amateurism in its best, original sense lies at the heart and soul of sportsmanship. Understanding good sportsmanship and practicing it in athletic competition prepare us for other, more important tests of character in life.

Everything that good sportsmanship means in practice flows in theory from a fundamental love and respect for the sport. You can't cheat or be a "bad sport," for example, and love the sport at the same time. And you can't put winning and personal gain above the Platonic ideal of a game well played and still be a "good sport."

But enough abstract moral philosophy; let's get down to cases:

• Sportsmanship means acting in a way that respects the spirit of the rules, as well the letter.

• Sportsmanship means not pouring it on when you are better than someone else at a game, but not patronizing him by slacking off, either.

• Sportsmanship is not arguing a call made by an opponent in a friendly contest without referees, even when it's clearly a bad one.

• Sportsmanship is winning *and* losing gracefully, and acting the same way toward your opponent whichever way it goes.

All this is tough, because we've been taught that winning is the *only* thing, a dictum that may be true in war but is preposterous when applied to a weekend softball game (or even the Super Bowl, for that matter). Being a good sport when you lose does not mean liking the fact that you lost; it does mean not letting on how much you hated it.

Okay, but how do you deal with a *bad* sport? The sort who calls every close one in his favor in a tennis match, who blames your good luck for his poor performance, who gloats over a win and whines about a loss. Easy: Stop playing with him. An adult who is a certified bad sport may be capable of being rehabilitated—one must cling to that straw, even if all experience in life contradicts it. But that doesn't mean you have to volunteer for the job.

STATIONERY

Most men would probably feel better if it were called writing paper or note cards or something. It's hard to avoid the fact that the word *stationery* conjures up an unwanted Christmas gift from an aunt you never liked much in the first place. But the fact is, you need stationery. Old office supplies are okay for some things—shopping lists or even letters to your parents if you're hoping that they'll send money—but for most occasions you'll need something at least marginally more ceremonial. Save the stuff with the smiling faces, golf slogans, and shamrocks for starting fires. You don't need to go nuts; just order a few supplies.

A stationery shop or good department store will fill you in on the hundreds of choices in size, color, type, weight, and the other accoutrements that the world of stationery involves, but the plain fact is that for every eventuality in your life you'll need two kinds of writing paper: informal and formal.

Formal sheets are the larger of the two—7 1/4 inches wide and 10 1/2 inches long is a good size—and both the sheet and the envelope should be imprinted with your name and address. The best color choice is white or off-white paper with fairly sober-looking black lettering. After all, this is what you'll be using for most of your personal correspondence, including condolence letters, so fuchsia trimmed in silver is definitely out.

For short notes—thank-yous, congratulations, birthday greetings—you'll want informal paper, and here you can use your imagination, provided you don't have too much of it. The sheets are smaller (6 1/4 inches by 8 inches), and they are usually folded. Here colors other than white are fine, but most people are happiest with beige, gray, pale blue, and other tame colors. (You'd be surprised how tired you can get of burgundy.) Again your name and address should be printed on the envelope, but the sheet should have just your name or perhaps just a monogram.

Something relatively new on the stationery front is the note card, which is just what it sounds like. It takes the place of the informal sheet, but it's smaller; so it's particularly good if you don't have a whole lot to say after you've said thank you for the swell present. Your name goes on the card, and your name and address are printed on the envelope. It's also fine as a gift card.

So where is your aunt now that you're ready for her?

Stand Up/Sit Down

The hoary dictum that a gentleman should always stand when a lady enters the room likely gave birth to the almost-as-ancient saw, "That was no lady, that was my wife," probably when some tired soul finally put his foot down in rebellion against an empty ritual. Think of it this way: If a person, lady or otherwise, wants all assembled to come to attention when she enters a room, she should earn it with her carriage, presentation, and style. It should come automatically only if she is a general or a queen.

In a restaurant. Two couples at a table, just settling into cocktails. A woman gets up (to go to the powder room, to call her bookie, whatever). What should a gentleman do? Stay put, unless she has to step over you to get out. All that pushing and shoving of chairs when a representative of one gender leaves and returns to a table looks plain dumb. Even if she's willing to reciprocate when you have to call Sportsphone, hopping up and down attracts undue attention to your table and disturbs the even distribution of martinis through your system. Sit.

In a living room. If it's a small party (fewer than ten people, say), rise as a new guest arrives. If it's a big party, hang on to your seat if you want to keep it.

In a business meeting. Are you kidding? Not for a female colleague, not these days, unless you want a scarlet "S" (for "sexist") branded on your forehead. But you *do* rise if visitors (of whatever sex) from outside the office enter the room and introductions are to be made. Then, everyone shakes hands before all are seated.

On a bus. These days, it's a judgment call. Old people and severely pregnant women deserve a break, but not just from seated men. Nowhere is it written that a seated woman cannot give up her seat to a sister with a compelling need for it. A man should not automatically bounce up just because the standee is female.

STREETWALKING

The essence of good form in changing times—and times are always changing—is that you follow rules of behavior that make sense and replace the ones that don't. But sometimes you hang on to a habit just because it still feels right, even though you know the rationale is obsolete.

The custom requiring the man to walk on the outside when strolling with a woman on a city street had its origins centuries ago, when people in upper floors disposed of their garbage by heaving it out the window. If the man was on the outside, he could presumably bear the brunt of the bombardment. Also, he could gallantly shield the lady from mud splashed up by carriages slogging though unpaved streets.

Garbage from on high is no longer a clear and present danger, and paved streets and horseless carriages have reduced the mud threat, so there's no longer any compelling reason for the man to station himself on the outside. But neither is there a *prima facie* case for an inside move, and the old way still looks right.

Stay put.

TABLE MANNERS

A mother gently removes a fistful of mashed potatoes from a baby's chubby little hand, replaces it with a spoon, clucks a loving word or two of encouragement, and—Eureka! Trumpet fanfare!!—the torch is passed to a new generation: Manners are born again.

All manners, social graces, and rules of etiquette flow philosophically from behavior learned at the table. That's why table manners used to be such a stern, no-nonsense business in genteel homes. Children were taught from a very early age to use correct utensils and were punished for using them incorrectly. If you picked up a fork when the implement of preference was a spoon, you were reprimanded. If you did it a second time, the voice of authority assumed its "final warning" tone. If you did it a third time, you were sent from the table without dessert, but only after finishing your peas.

Everything else followed logically. "Please" pass the mashed potatoes/"Thank you" for passing them. Keep your elbows off the table. Don't slouch. Eat slowly and quietly. Don't interrupt. Honor thy father and thy mother. *Ad infinitum,* or until you grew up and moved out, whichever came first.

The payoff for such rigidity would not come until years later, when a young suitor was put to the test of fire: Sunday dinner at his girlfriend's home. If he had learned his long-ago lessons well, his table manners would pass muster, and there would be some basis other than a young girl's infatuation for bestowing tentative parental approval on him.

But the price was high, too high, it must have seemed to a post–World War II generation of parents whose psyches had been rapped along with their knuckles once too often. Whatever the reason, the pendulum started to swing away from the hard school of table manners, and it kept on going. Autocracy at the dinner table, practicioners of the old ways observed in horror, gave way to anarchy, to the point that a new generation of parents abdicated their responsibility and permitted their kids to eat any which way. And so it came to pass that the way a person held his or her fork became symbol and metaphor to doomsayers everywhere of the impending decline and fall of Western civilization.

Okay, maybe table manners didn't go all the way to hell in a handbasket, but it is true that the generations born after midcentury seem to have been less rigidly schooled in dining etiquette, and as a consequence many young adults today may be confused about what rules, if any, to follow.

Well, we have good news. Don't worry about having to sign up for that night course in remedial table manners. Put aside thoughts of long, dreary weekends spent doing research on proper utensil selection. There is, we are happy to report, but one and only one utterly absolute rule that you need to know pertaining to manners at the table. Tucking your napkin under your chin, reaching across three plates for the salt, starting before others have been served, saucering your coffee, and certainly eating with the wrong utensil—all the traditional table sins can be forgiven, save one. Ready? Listen carefully: DO NOT TALK WITH YOUR MOUTH FULL OR CHEW WITH YOUR MOUTH OPEN.

You may want to call that two rules instead of one, but whatever you do, don't break it (or them), and you'll pass muster in our house. Of course, if you want to go beyond the bare minimum, you can take few additional positive steps. You can wait until everybody is served before starting to eat. You can pick out someone who seems to know what he (but usually she) is doing at a dinner party and follow his (or her) lead in utensil selection and use. You can ask that things be passed to you instead of reaching across the table for them. You can even call your mother before going out to eat and ask for a quick refresher course on some of the things that she was taught when she was growing up. But you needn't get bent out of shape about anything so long as you DO NOT TALK WITH YOUR MOUTH FULL OR CHEW WITH YOUR MOUTH OPEN.

This seems to be as good a time as any for a brief disquisition on "boardinghouse reach," a term that shows the linkage between table and other kinds of manners. The term was used as a social slur with a specific commentary on a person's table manners. The upper classes, after all, did not live in boardinghouses. To say that someone had boardinghouse reach meant that he was common, or at least of a lower social order, and not only that he reached half the length of the table to grab the gravy. We bother to digress because, with the disappearance of boardinghouses for people to practice their reach in, it won't be long before no one will know what the term means, and it will fall out of the language entirely.

There are also a few problem foods that can give you fits if you aren't forearmed. Among them:

Lobster. No problem, just don't eat it anywhere but Maine, and there only outdoors, on a pier, in a swimsuit.

Chili. Wear a lobster bib.

Snails. Never order anything that requires a special tool. Also, there are many easier ways to eat a lot of garlic and butter.

Soup. Silence is golden. Dip the spoon away from you, lean over slightly, don't slurp, and never tilt your bowl to get the last spoonful (unless you're eating lunch at a good diner).

Barbecued ribs. The only place they're likely to be any good is at a bona fide barbecue joint, where no one cares what your face and fingers look like after you finish, so eat them any way you please . . . just as long as you DO NOT TALK WITH YOUR MOUTH FULL OR CHEW WITH YOUR MOUTH OPEN.

TACT

What's that? You don't know exactly what tact is? That's understandable. It's much underemployed these days and definitely has an old-fashioned ring to it. But that probably means it has some deep-seated value, so don't turn this page.

Think of tact as a fine line between a hard truth and a soft lie, and accept the fact that it's a modern moral imperative to live close to the line. If a caveman didn't like the look or smell of a stranger, he could (a) knock his block off, or (b) move to the next mountain in open disgust. Civilized man, no matter how disapproving he might be of another passenger on Spaceship Earth, is (or ought to be) impelled to exercise a modicum of tact.

To wit:

• Instead of demanding to see a colleague's high school diploma if he doesn't grasp a strategy that you've just explained with abundant lucidity, say something about how tough the concept is and go back over it step by step.

• Instead of suggesting to a friend with a new haircut that she can always wear a wig until it grows out, say that she's the only person you know besides Grace Jones who could carry off that style.

• Instead of spitting out the creamed okra when your host leaves the table to fetch more, say something nice about the jellied succotash.

• Instead of saying the breakup was all her fault, say it was all your fault.

Tact means not prying (and that includes not asking leading questions). It means letting someone else reveal confidences or raise sensitive subjects without comment, but not doing either yourself. Tact means holding back in those instances where the truth hurts and withholding it won't make matters worse by misleading anyone. Most of all, tact means distance. That distance will vary according to how well you know someone, but even the best of friends won't take kindly to your tromping around in their emotions without a specific invitation.

TAKING HER OUT TO A BALLGAME

Y ou've met each other's friends, spent a weekend together in the country, and started talking about a spring vacation in Paris. You've negotiated peace terms concerning Japanese food, Fassbinder films, and Rodney Dangerfield. You're now ready for the next big step in your relationship—taking her to a sporting event.

Short of meeting her parents, introducing the special woman in your life to your favorite spectator sport may be the most traumatic challenge you have to face as an adult male engaged in the mating game. The key word, of course, is *spectator*—these days a woman is every bit as likely as a man to love participant sports. But it's still rare to find a woman who's lived and died (mostly died) with the Cubs since she was seven years old, or who has never missed a TV minute of a single Super Bowl game, or who believes a college hoops tournament is the best possible way to spend the Christmas holiday.

So if you're the sort of person in whose psyche a deep and unquestioning love of a particular sport took firm root almost before conscious memory, there are a number of basic guidelines to follow when introducing it to a person who is, after all, a relative newcomer to your life.

Examine your motives. Are you really looking for another pal to go to games with? What if she doesn't like it? More important, what if she does? Are you ready to share this particular piece of your inner life? Is this a test? If so, is it a final exam? (If your answer to the last question isn't no, then maybe you should reconsider and go to the movies.)

Go first class. Your idea of heaven may be a few hot dogs, a gang of cold beers, and a bleacher seat among "fans who really know the game." (Translation: They'll fight over anything.) But for first-timers, a proper lunch or dinner at a smart restaurant before the event and the best seats you can put your hands on are *de rigueur*. Always give it your best shot.

Examine first principles. Your pre-game meal together will give you the opportunity to explain what it is about the sport that really appeals to you. Your goal should be to have her understand your harmless passion, even if she's not destined to share it. This is also an occasion for introspection, and you may be surprised what you learn about yourself. Is it the brilliant skating and deft stick handling that attract you to hockey? Or its incipient violence? Either is okay, but you should know for sure, and having to explain it to her may help you learn.

Don't stack the deck. Pick an "average" game or match if it's her introduction to the sport. If she wants to leave at halftime just because it's 10 degrees Fahrenheit and she's not keen on risking frostbite to learn the difference between a flea flicker and a fly pattern, your relationship will suffer, particularly if it's a playoff game, your dearly beloveds are two-point underdogs, and you've bet a bundle at even money just to show faith. You've already got all the pressure you can handle, so take someone else to the big games until you establish that she genuinely likes the sport.

Don't come on like Howard Cosell. Resist the natural temptation to show off how much you know about the finer points of the game. You'll certainly sound patronizing, and she's not likely to be impressed. Stick to answering questions when asked. And if you must offer a little color commentary, do it *sotto voce*—there's nothing more boring than a sports bore.

Be flexible. What if your own very first basketball game had been between two teams who favored the zone defense and the four-corners offense? Even though the very idea is foreign to your soul, be prepared to leave early if it's clear that your companion is bored to tears. Of this you can be certain: A seventeen-inning pitchers' duel can kill a romance quicker than infidelity. Cut your losses and go home when she begins to nod off.

Leave the competition to the competitors. If it turns out that her knowledge of the sport is greater than you expected, don't take it as a threat to your manhood. Rejoice. Most of all, do not act like your team has just lost the Big Game.

Be a good sport. You have to be prepared for the possibility that no matter how sensitively you've presented it, the woman of your dreams may not cotton to the sport that has possessed you since you were Beaver's age. She may even flat-out hate it. If that happens, there's nothing you can do but shrug and take it like a man. Be mature. Be cool. After all, there are other fish in the sea.

TAKING YOUR LEAVE

There are two things to know about leave-taking—how to sense when your hosts are ready for everyone to go home and how to slip away unnoticed when you are but they aren't.

The first is easy enough—the offering of coffee is a sure sign that you should start thinking about where you put your coat; clearing away party debris means you should put it on. Hang around for the gaping yawns and flickering of the lights only if you are (a) an especially close friend of the hosts, (b) are having a great time, or (c) think you are in love with another late stayer. Preferably all three.

(When you are the host, don't be afraid to send late stayers on their way with a hearty "Last call!" and a joggle of the light switch. Just be sure enough about your relations with your guests to count on laughter rather than embarrassed silence in response. And you may not want to try it if your boss is in the middle of a long joke.)

Taking leave *before* the party's over is at best tricky, and at a dinner party, impossible (unless you're a convincing actor and are willing to fake food poisoning). Half an hour after dessert and coffee is the earliest you can make your getaway.

Follow this rule of thumb—the bigger the party, the easier it is to spring yourself without hurting anyone's feelings. Say it's a large gathering. Not cocktails, where there's always a dinner engagement as an excuse to leave early, but a gala that starts at 9:00 and is expected to sail into the wee hours. You don't want to offend your hosts, but you're not up to a long evening of first names and blurred faces, of shouting to be heard by someone you don't want to talk to in the first place, of too much smoke and too little ventilation.

The solution? The 15-Minute Sweep. Zero in on your hosts from the moment you enter (*circa* 9:30). If there are two of them, most likely they'll be working separately. Stick with one, then the other until each has to go off to do hostly things. Then work your way steadily around the room(s). Clockwise or counter-clockwise, it doesn't matter (too bad if it did—a recent study confirmed a growing number of people born into the digital age don't know the difference). Untouched drink in hand (you don't want to get too comfortable), nod greetings to everyone you recognize. Don't tarry to talk, though; your mission is to be seen, not heard. Work your way back toward the front door. As soon as the coast is clear, you're history.

Obviously, this won't be easy if the party's on the shy side of 50 in number, or if it's the dead of winter and your coat gets carted away and hidden. But it will work more often than you think. The reason for that, of course, is also the sobering downside of the ploy's success—one's presence is never missed quite so much as one might hope.

The next day, call to thank your host(s) for a wonderful evening, and in doing so scope out whether your early departure drew notice. Chances are at least 3 to 1 that it didn't, but if it did, be ready to claim a sudden feeling of nausea as the reason for your abrupt and early exit. No one ever argues with nausea.

TEA

Tea is something one "takes" (not "drinks," although you do that as well in the taking of it) when on vacation in the United Kingdom. It's an excuse to eat scones, cookies, pastries, and sandwiches with their crusts trimmed, and to do it between meals. It's often "high," though no alcohol is ever served. It's typically served at 4:00 p.m., when all but the idle rich are hard at work. It's related to Tea Dancing, which takes place later in the afternoon *before* cocktails, if you can believe it. It's something that avant garde heavy hitters in commerce and industry have taken to "taking" instead of booze and salted nuts at the same posh business-district hotels where meals called "power breakfasts" are served earlier in the day. It's so falsely familiar to most Americans (that is, we know what tea is, without having a clue what *tea* means) that we can well understand why Winston Churchill said that the Americans and the British were two peoples divided by a common language. But it's also something that the likes of Alec Guinness, Laurence Olivier, Albert Finney, Michael Caine, and Sean Connery "take," and look pretty swell in the doing, thank you. Maybe there's something to this tea thing after all.

TELEPHONES

So much of modern life spent on the telephone, so little written about good phone form. Until now.

• You're in her living room, she's in the kitchen whipping up an intimate supper for two, the phone rings, she asks you to answer it—and a man's voice at the other end of the line asks to speak to her. "May I tell her who's calling?" is fine for the office, but out of bounds here (so, by the way, was your "Hello"—you should have answered "Mary Smith's residence" in your most cultured, butlerlike voice). "One moment, please" is the correct response, unless she's hand-beating the Hollandaise, in which case "Could you call back in fifteen minutes?" will do the trick. "May I take a message" might seem more polite, but she may not want you to know the names of other male callers.

• Unless you're absolutely, one-hundred-percent certain of another person's waking/sleeping schedule, never call between the hours of 10:00 p.m. and 9:00 a.m. We all deserve a respite from the telephone.

• Always ask the person you're calling if this is a good time to talk before launching into your 15-minute monologue on the trade-deficit problem. Who knows, she might be busy folding socks.

• Say a friend is feeling chatty, you're not, and you want to cut short the conversation without being rude. You can concoct an emergency—"I really must be going, the cat is on fire"—but it's better to mix equal parts of truth and white lie, and promise to make amends. As in, "I want to talk about this some more, but I have a splitting headache. Can I call you back in a couple of hours/days/years?"

• Never break up on the telephone. It may seem the easy way, but it's also the coward's way.

• We're nearing the 21st century, and machines are here to stay, so when you reach an answering machine (see ANSWERING MACHINES), leave a message, for goodness' sake! Who do you think is the loser if you take the "I never talk to machines" approach? Grow up.

THANK YOU

Captain Kangaroo and Mr. Greenjeans were right all along—Please and Thank You *are* the two most important words in the English language. (Okay, *three,* but who's counting?)

If you remember to say "Please pass the salt," "May I speak to her, please?," "One black coffee, please," and "Yes, please," that just about covers the waterfront on Please. But there's a little more ritual attached to Thank You.

Some people think thank-you notes are for girls. You can't blame them entirely, since for some reason it's the bride who always writes thank-you notes for wedding presents. (Or used to, before grooms came to their liberated senses and started sharing the chore fifty-fifty.) And who ever heard of a Dad forcing anyone to write to an Aunt Sally to thank her for the velour play shirt she sent? But some of us don't have wives, so let's start with the basics: When someone does something nice for you, you should say thank you. We'd like to think that there are more nice things than we could possibly list, but the things that require acknowledgment tend to fall into categories—a gift, a meal, a ticket, a bed for the night (see BREAD-AND-BUTTER GIFTS).

You can say thank you over the phone, but a telephone call can be more trouble than it's worth in some ways—you might be interrupting someone, maybe no one is home, or maybe you're just getting a busy signal. No, we vote for the thank-you note. It will cost you precisely 22 cents and about two minutes. Moreover, you can write it at your convenience, and the recipient—unaccustomed as he or she is to dealing with the sort of gentleman you manifestly are—will be pleasantly surprised and pleased.

It doesn't really matter what you write on (although elsewhere we pretend that it does; see STATIONERY), or even what your message is (so long as it's grammatical). Say that you love the tie or that the dinner party was a delight or that you never knew Cleveland was so great until she showed you the sights. A postdate note saying "thanks for the terrific night" has been know to reduce the supposedly crusty Eighties woman to chocolate pudding.

Emily Post notwithstanding, there's no trick to saying thank you except saying it.

TIPPING

Tipping is troublesome and awkward for a lot of American men, and for a lot of pretty good reasons. It seems to belong to an old-world, class-conscious society that we supposedly rebelled against once upon a time in our mythical history. It doesn't quite square with the "honest day's work for an honest day's pay" adage. Insofar as there is uncertainty built into the practice (how much? who gets one? who doesn't?), it is a source of some anxiety. Most of us would probably prefer having the remuneration of those who serve us be determined by someone else (a service charge? an adequate wage?), because it's a lot easier than making individual judgment calls on a case-by-case basis.

And yet, when a total stranger comes up to you at a hotel's registration desk, picks up the small suitcase and briefcase you carried in yourself, and guides you down a clearly marked hall to your room, you let him do it—and you give him money. You tip him for this totally unnecessary service because that's the way he makes his living. It doesn't *feel* particularly right, but it's the right thing to do.

Even when the service is essential—when you have a lot of heavy luggage that you can't handle by yourself—it would still *feel* better to have a charge for his services built into your room's cost rather than have to tabulate an acceptable sum (a buck a bag? more? a little extra if he's particularly helpful, or just pleasant?) to pay out on the spot.

But that's not the way it is; tipping is the way it is. So come on, stop grumbling, and learn some ground rules for appropriate behavior in an imperfect part of life.

TOO MUCH

At first blush, gross overtipping seems to be one of those self-created problems that wouldn't be a problem at all if you didn't worry about it yourself. Who really cares if you tip far more than the going rate? Certainly not the cabdrivers, waiters, and bell-men on the receiving end. Restaurant owners don't much like flagrant overtippers, whose mere presence can cause the staff to get giddy and greedy and neglectful of regular customers. But that aside, what harm does it do?

None, really, but it can make the perpetrator look like a nou-veau jerk who flaunts his wealth to seem bigger than he is, or an insecure creature who believes he can buy acceptance and re-spect. We'd even suggest that tipping way over customary norms upsets a carefully constructed social balance—if such a sugges-tion weren't so vacuous.

Fact is, there's nothing whatever wrong with a little moderate overtipping—20 percent instead of 15 percent, an extra 50 cents plus taxi fare and tip, two bucks per bag at the airport's curbside luggage check if it's a cold day. It spreads the sunshine, and no one's going to give you a hard time, least of all us.

TOO LITTLE

Undertipping *is* a problem because it's flat-out unfair to other people. Occasional undertippers are usually just ignorant; chronic undertippers are just plain cheapskates. We're talking here about situations where the service has been average to better-than-average, not where poor service has been rewarded accordingly. Undertippers of the chronic sort typically try to rationalize their cheapness; the merely ignorant, of course, are blissfully unaware that they are doing anything untoward.

We say elsewhere (see MONEY) that you could do a lot worse than go through life paying a little more than your share. That's certainly true when it comes to tipping. Keep in mind that you have probably more to start with than the people who are per-forming the personal services that, according to custom, call for gratuities.

If you have a stingy streak, direct it toward people who are richer than you are. They can afford it.

NOTHING AT ALL

Stiffing is altogether different from undertipping. It's a serious act, never to be undertaken lightly, that is, on exceedingly rare occasions, the only appropriate course of action.

Extreme and repeated rudeness, gross negligence despite cautionary warnings, utter failure to respond to a reasonable request for service—there are times when nothing will get the correct signal across except . . . nothing. Please note that this short list of justifications for stiffing does *not* include bad food at a restaurant (unless the waiter cooked it) or a noisy, dirty, uncomfortable room in a hotel (unless the bellman owns it). You only stiff a person for utterly failing, without sufficient reason, to fulfill his or her mutually understood obligations to you. After all, when was the last time your boss docked you because he didn't like your work?

In using the following general guide to tipping, keep in mind a couple of caveats: The customary tip for similar services varies from region to region (not to mention from country to country), so always ask about local practice if you are uncertain; and the figures given here are for "average" service. Sorry, we can't be more precise than that. So stiff us.

Accommodations: Hotels, Motels, Inns

Doorman. One dollar for taking bags out of the car. Fifty cents for calling a cab, one dollar if he has to work to get one.

Bellman. One dollar per bag; more if they're very heavy.

Room service. Fifteen percent of the bill. If there is a service charge listed on the bill, this doesn't take the place of a tip.

Garage (valet parking). One dollar each time the car is brought up (50 cents in smaller cities).

Maid. Leave a tip of one dollar per room per day at the end of the stay and more if they've provided a special service.

Restaurants

Bartender. Ten to 15 percent for drinks ordered at the bar before you sit down.

Waiter. Fifteen percent; more for excellent service.

Captain. Five percent. Tip him in person as you leave or specify the amount on the charge slip.

Cellar master/wine steward. Two to five dollars or 10 percent of wine cost if he's been particularly helpful. Tip him in person as you leave.

Maître d'. It's certainly not necessary to tip him, but it's a good idea if you're a regular or want to be remembered when you return. Five dollars and up, depending on how fancy the restaurant; tip him in person as you leave.

Coat check. One dollar for one coat; for more than one, 50 cents per coat.

Washroom attendant. Fifty cents, minimum.

Travel

Airline or train porter. One dollar per bag.

Taxi. Fifteen percent for most trips. Up to 20 percent for above-average comfort or driving skill, or if driver handles luggage for you or stops and waits while you run an errand.

Limousine. Fifteen to 20 percent.

Apartments

Everyone who provides service throughout the year should be tipped at Christmas, with the amount depending on the size of the maintenance staff and how much time they spent helping you.

Superintendent. Thirty to forty dollars; less if there's a handyman who does repairs.

Handyman. Ten to twenty dollars.

Doorman. Twenty to thirty dollars.

Elevator operator. Ten dollars.

Services

Hair care. Fifteen percent at the barbershop. In a salon: Ten percent to the haircutter; one dollar to the person who shampoos your hair, two dollars if he/she blow-dries it; one dollar to the manicurist. Don't tip the owner.

Shoeshine. Fifty cents.

Parking. One dollar.

TOAST

This has traditionally been a man's job, and that's our tough luck, because it's lonely standing up there in front of a lot of raised glasses at a formal dinner party, waiting for an attack of inspired eloquence. "Over the teeth/Past the gums/Watch out stomach/Here it comes" may earn a patronizing chuckle or two, but it really won't do if you're the best man at a wedding or a guest at a special dinner party. On the other hand, a proper toast—one that *is* inspired and eloquent, not to mention pithy and pointed—is tough work, and it's no wonder that each of us has heard a dozen bad ones for every good one to come down the pike.

Fortunately you will have time to prepare; the occasions where one might be expected to offer a toast are usually not impromptu get-togethers. And prepare you should, because this is one time where it is definitely bad form to be at a loss for words.

Sex, Money, Religion, and Politics—the four most important topics of civilized conversation—are out of bounds for toasts unless sufficiently denatured to guarantee against divisiveness. This is the time for praise, sentimentality, wit, expressing gratitude. Be ready to elevate an occasion with a well-crafted compliment. Pick another setting to reopen an old debate.

Sports metaphors are okay, as are references to history, the classics, music, and the arts—assuming, of course, that the reference is apt. For example, you shouldn't gas on about how the toastee's leadership qualities remind you of Patton if he (or she) happens to be an ardent pacifist. Showing off a bit is fine, but only if your remarks stay on the mark.

Recalling a story from a childhood association, or describing your first meeting, or revealing a little-known fact about the person being toasted can be effective, so long as it leads to the point, and quickly. Ditto a telling quotation from a favorite author, so long as it's short enough to be memorized and delivered without note cards. (Unless you are a high school English teacher, this may be the only time in your adult life that you'll have an opportunity to quote from a poem in public. Just make sure it's not one of Rod McKuen's).

How long a toast should be depends on when it's delivered. At a dinner party, when there is food on the plates, figure one minute tops. But with brandy and coffee, or at a stand-up reception, you can go on for a while. Don't, however, get so caught up in your own erudition and wordsmanship that you trigger the MEGO Effect among your audience. (MEGO, of course, stands for "My Eyes Glaze Over.")

Practice in front of a mirror, and time yourself. Sounds dopey, but when was the last time you gave a formal speech in public? Chances are it was in eighth-grade speech class, but even if you were a world-class high school debater, a little practice makes a lot of sense.

Speed-readers who zipped ahead looking for a few perfect toasts to crib will be disappointed. You won't find any here, because a good toast must perforce be tailor-made for the occasion. Indeed, the more personal and pointed a toast is, the better it's likely to be received, so a pre-fab model would be of spurious value.

But we will tell you of one toast, or a fragment of one, that we heard a long time ago, and which has worn well. It was delivered at a small wedding by the best man, a college professor who warned before he started that he was accustomed to speaking for 50 minutes at a clip. He said nice words about the bride, and about the groom, and then said that what made the event so special was the love for them both that brought everyone together in celebration. And then he proposed a toast to harmony, and specifically "to all our best qualities."

The vicissitudes of modern life being what they are, the marriage has not survived. But the toast, with its affirmation of humanity, has.

Cheers! Here's to all our best qualities!

VALENTINE'S DAY

The dumbest holiday in the book—in our book, at least—
is St. Valentine's Day.

Consider, for starters, the story of the saint it honors.
(Actually, a number of fellows named Valentine achieved saint-
hood; it must have been a more popular name a long time ago.
But that's another story. Or stories.)

He—Valentine the First—was a priest and physician during
the third century A.D. in Rome (not a Catholic priest, but a prac-
titioner of one of the officially sanctioned state religions in the
Roman Empire) who was imprisoned in the year 270 for protect-
ing early Christians from persecution. While in jail he converted
to Christianity and, even more impressive, restored the sight of
his jailer's blind daughter. You'd think that would have earned
him time off for good behavior, but he was clubbed to death for
his troubles. Sure, he became a saint, but he'd probably have
settled for parole.

So what, you might well ask, does St. Valentine's sad fate
have to do with the romantic aura and social customs we associ-
ate with the celebration of his Day? Zip. Zero. *Nada.* Absolutely
nothing. For *their* origins you have to go back a few more centuries still, to *really* ancient Rome, for a short history lesson.

The Lupercal is the spot where Romulus and Remus were
sucked by a wolf (Lupercal/lupus/lobo/wolf; it all hangs together)
so they could grow up and found Rome. An annual festival called
the Lupercalia came to be held there every February 15 (No, no
one knows exactly when the first one took place, but it had to be
after Romulus and Remus were weaned) to honor the god Lupercus. Now, *he* was the Lycian analogue to the ancient Greek
god Pan, and his (Lupercus'/Pan's) job was to protect the Ro-
mans' flocks from wolves by playing his flute. Not all wolves were
good wolves, you see.

Huh?! What does a bunch of people having a party in the middle of February have to do with little Hallmark cupids? Well, say

the "experts," you see, ahhh, the thing is, mid-February is also the beginning of the mating season for birds, so maybe . . .

Hold it right there. You want the truth? *They don't know.* "They" cite references to birds mating on St. Valentine's day in Chaucer and Shakespeare, but *no one knows* for sure why February 14 came to be linked with bad candy in heart-shaped boxes. And somewhere it got lost in the shuffle that the ancient Roman celebration was really a *fertility* festival, not an exaltation of romantic love. Think about the difference for a minute.

Fertility and murder, that's what Valentine's Day is all about, if you count the 1929 massacre of seven bootleggers from Bugs Moran's gang by their counterparts from Al Capone's. Nothing much else worthy of note has ever happened on February 14, unless you feel strongly about the birthdays of Copernicus, Jimmy Hoffa, and/or Florence Henderson.

There, that's out of our system, but we're still left with the problem of what to do about Valentine's Day. One thing *not* to do is be the first on your block to rip the mask off V.D.—takes on a whole different feel if you think of it that way, doesn't it?— by actually refusing to buy a gift, card, or both for your sweetheart. It needs to be revealed for the big, fat, historical humbug it is, but let someone else be a martyr. Remember where it got St. Valentine.

No, it won't do to go *mano a mano* with anything that's gotten to be such a big deal. Of the seven billion greeting cards Americans buy each year, fully 850 million are Valentines of one sort or another. And the candy industry racks up $570 million in sales of sweets for sweethearts on Valentine's Day. And now that the rose has been officially anointed by Congress and the President as America's Flower, it will certainly continue to be the posy of preference on February 14: Sixty-five million roses (red is the favorite color) are delivered on Valentine's Day.

The question, then, is not *whether* to acknowledge Valentine's Day, but *how* to acknowledge it with grace, flair, and a modicum of dignity. Here are four suggestions:

1. A perfect rose with fresh morning coffee and orange juice

that you've squeezed yourself, all brought to her in bed on a tray (some clichés come in handy);

2. Dinner at an unabashedly romantic restaurant, where you can actually hold hands and not feel foolish (but do avoid establishments with strolling musicians, unless life for you is a 1940s movie);

3. A brief note, written on just about anything *except* a Valentine's Day card (i.e., no hearts, no cupids, no printed sentiments—sorry, Hallmark), delivered to her office or left on her pillow;

4. A distinctive but not breathtakingly expensive gift, something decidedly personal (i.e., no toaster ovens), and not candy (sorry, Godiva). Think old silver.

One final word: If you are over the age of 21, do not send a Valentine's Day card to your mother unless you first clear it with your analyst.

WARDROBE

How did this happen? One minute the choice is button-down or not and the next minute they're suggesting that men would be a lot cooler in the summer if they wore skirts. But do you panic? You do not. You sit back, watch *Miami Vice,* and consider the Well-Dressed Man.

It would be simple if men could spend all their time in black tie. Guys happen to look astonishingly attractive in a tuxedo, and that's a fact. True, it takes a little time getting the tie just right, but it's worth it (see BLACK TIE). But what about the rest of the time, when rental is not a viable alternative?

Dressing well is as complex as you want it to be. If you're invigorated by the prospect of experimenting with different looks and challenged by the new fabrics, you can run along to the Armani show. If you're still not sure why you need two pairs of shoes since you can wear only one pair at a time, you're what's called a *tabula rasa* and can use a little help.

First, an important distinction. A Moneyed Gentleman has one of everything in every color and an extra for the stables, but chances are you're a Working Gentlemen. That may grate, but there it is.

Here's what a Working Gentleman needs to look his best, starting with the inner you.

Underwear. Clark Gable didn't need an undershirt, and it's been a long time since Marlon Brando looked good in one, so we say to hell with them. Boxers or briefs? Hey, we're too smart to get dragged into that one. We will say this, however—your underwear should never be so outlandish as to trigger uncontrollable laughter in a hospital emergency room.

Socks. Except for handkerchiefs, this is the dullest clothing—or at least should be. White for sports, and black, brown, or blue the rest of the time, depending on the color of your pants, except for those *(rare!)* moments when it's argyles or bust. And for God's sake, make sure they're long enough.

Dress shirts. This (and in ties) is where you can get a little reckless, provided you keep your wits about you. Don't, for instance, buy any dress shirt with short sleeves. Avoid black shirts—who needs the pressure? Do get as much cotton in the shirt as possible. And take advantage of anyone in the clothing store who looks sharp to you for advice on what patterns and colors got together.

Suits. The Cardinal Suit Rule is as follows: Figure out the most you can pay for your suits and then pay at least $100 more. It will show. The Second Suit Rule: Buy as many as you can afford and then buy one more. If you can have only one per season, make them a darkish gray, medium-weight wool two piece (vests are like tonsils, totally unnecessary) and a khaki-colored cotton suit. Every shirt, tie, and sweater ever made will go with them. If you're feeling playful, try corduroy in the winter and seersucker in the summer. We remain skeptical about wash-and-wear suits and unalterably opposed to polyester.

Casual shirts. Feel free to wear short sleeves, and don't be shy about colors or prints or anything. If your friends don't like your polo player or alligator or whatever, get new friends or a pair of scissors.

Slacks. Who the hell invented beltless trousers? We say that any pants worth wearing are worth holding up with a belt. We do move with the times, though, embracing bell-bottoms, pleats, pegged pants, even balloon pants in their time, provided that they're in colors that you can see before you hear them. Even so, we believe that a well-dressed man does not make a big production out of the wearing of trousers. He is happy to be seen in gray, blue, brown, camel hair or tweed; wool, corduroy, or cotton, no matter the weather or the occasion. When he is off duty, he wears chinos or jeans.

Jackets. Have as many sports coats as you can get your hands on, but settle for ones in camel hair, tweed, and corduroy if closet space is tight. The Blue Blazer Controversy rages on, and a good case can be made for not wearing one anywhere except at the America's Cup. If it feels good, do it. But no cap, please. And no plaids. Ever.

Belts. A boring but necessary accessory. You should own a black and a brown belt for most occasions, and you are allowed to have one frivolous belt. If you've visited the Southwest, for instance, you no doubt have a belt with your name burned into it and adorned with a huge Texas belt buckle. Go ahead—wear it with your jeans. Maybe no one will see you.

Suspenders. Good on the right man. Just be sure it's you.

Ties. They cut off your circulation and attract spaghetti sauce, but let's face it—they're here to stay. Sometimes it seems as if there's only one tie out there, yellow with red markings. But if you put your mind to it, you can (and should) branch out. Every man needs a red tie for courage, a polka-dot tie for style, a paisley tie for tradition, and a striped tie for job interviews. When you buy a tie, keep in mind the shirt(s) and suit(s) you're planning to wear it with. After all, your tie and shirts are what lend your suit its diversity. Stick with cotton, wool, or silk and try not to keep buying the same one over and over again.

Shoes. Some folks say that shoes are the first thing apt to be noticed about a well-dressed man; others insist they should be inconspicuous. We say they should be as expensive as you can manage and as comfortable as is humanly possible. Two pairs of tie shoes (make them brown and black—oxblood is for the insecure) and a pair of loafers should give you happy feet. Buckles are out, but tassles are okay. Suede brogues are perfect if you're planning to become the squire of an English manor. If we were Fred Astaire (and on good days we think we are), we'd suggest you get some patent leather dancing shoes for black-tie affairs.

Sweaters. Women love a man in a sweater, and who are we to disagree with them? Save the bulky ones for the slopes, though. An urban gentleman wears thin wool or cashmere sweaters and vests in all shapes and styles, plus cotton for late spring and early fall. Bright colors and patterns should be handled with caution; don't forget that loud sweaters are Jerry Lewis's trademark.

Raincoats. Surprisingly dull, despite the fact that they cost so much. In the South this is the only coat you need, but just because it has to do double duty, don't feel you need to get one that makes a fashion statement. North or South, beige, black, blue, gray, or army-green will do nicely, thank you. And always a plain lining, please.

Overcoats. So it's not raining, but it is cold. You've got lots of choices here, and they're all quite pleasant. Stay with a dark color—gray or black—and don't get carried away with tailoring or buckles or epaulettes. It's hard to imagine a situation or a planet in which gray herringbone is not absolutely appropriate. Leather overcoats are for rock stars, pimps, and drug dealers.

Pajamas. If for no other reason, you should keep them around so that women you admire can model the oversize tops. Most men sleep in pajamas only when they suspect that there will be a fire in the middle of the night. And even then, only soft cotton ones in solid colors.

Bathrobes. These are another story, and a mighty provocative one at that. Bathrobes aren't essential, but they can make you feel like Paul Newman or the star of *Falcon Crest,* whoever that might be. Terrycloth is nice, but it's for hanging on the back of the bathroom door. When a proper gentleman receives in his bathrobe, he wears silk or polished cotton, and he drinks his Scotch neat. That goes for you, too, even if you prefer bourbon.

By the way, seersucker and velour are not the same as silk and cotton. Just ask Paul Newman.

Resort wear. It really isn't necessary to buy a new wardrobe when you go on vacation. You shouldn't have to wear silly clothes just to sip drinks with little umbrellas in them, and you always have your golf and tennis stuff to fall back on for *gauche.* We find that just about anything a fellow can't do in chinos and a polo shirt doesn't bear doing. But then there's the question of shorts. Say what you will about shorts, it all comes down to this: If you've got the legs for 'em, go for it. If not, act high-handed and say that shorts are only for English boys in boarding school. When choosing a bathing suit, try not to look like a beach boy out of *Night of the Iguana*. Tom Selleck doesn't flaunt it. Why should you?

Accessories. A good watch and one set of great (but elegantly simple) cuff-links. Beyond that, you're courting fashion disaster.

Bibliography. If you take clothing seriously, and we believe you should, you may want more guidance than a manners book can provide. We recommend *Man At His Best: The Esquire Guide to Style,* by the Editors of *Esquire* magazine. Surprised?

WEDDING

If the soul of a society is truly revealed in its private and public ceremonies, then our times might well be called the Regency Period of American history. Consider the style in which people get married these days.

A couple of decades back (were the Sixties really so long ago?), a young bride and groom might simply head for the nearest park or hilltop in the country, exchange garlands of flowers, and pledge to live together in peace, while friends sang protest songs and strummed guitars and smoked funny cigarettes. Make love, not war.

Fast forward to today. Engraved invitations, engagement parties, bridal showers and bachelor parties, formal rehearsal dinners, cadres of ushers and bridesmaids, hundreds of guests, limousines, and gala receptions complete with dance bands. In case you haven't been married recently, be advised that the Big Wedding is back.

This is not, from a curmudgeon's perspective, an altogether Good Thing. To observe families of middle-class and even more modest means spending thousands, even tens-of-thousands of dollars on a nuptial extravaganza makes one suspect that a certain madness has descended on the land. Hasn't anyone read any statistics on divorce lately? Isn't anyone a little queasy about investing so much time, energy, and family resources on what looks to be, at best, a fifty-fifty chance of Forever? And setting hard-headed realism aside in favor of unbridled romanticism, isn't there a clear and present danger with the Big Wedding of permitting the pomp to dominate the circumstance? Is love really blind?

Enough quibbling. The fact is, a young man who gets married these days must be ready for the whole nine yards, from high-level negotiations on the wedding date that would put the SALT talks to shame, to back-alley fights over how many friends his parents can invite (never enough/always too many, depending on whose mother is asked), to whether his attendants' cummerbunds must, absolutely *must,* match the color of her bridesmaids' dresses. Details, details. Enough policy decisions to keep the entire executive branch of a medium-sized country working full-tilt for six months. And virtually infinite opportunities for inter-family warfare (just wait until her mother tells your mother where the rehearsal dinner should be held).

So what did you expect? Bliss? That comes later. For the half month or so before a Big Wedding, every day holds all the promise of a dental appointment. Unless . . . unless you play your cards right, bow to tradition, thank your lucky stars, stand in front of the mirror, and read this aloud: "It's Not *My* Job."

That's right, it's not *your* job. It's *hers.* No matter that you're both ardent feminists, or that your relationship is based on sharing and mutual respect, or that you both despise sexual stereotyping. When it comes to the Big Wedding, the woman is in charge. No ifs, ands, or buts. And if you doubt it for a minute, just try telling her what kind of flowers the bridesmaids ought to carry.

You should be "consulted" on all important matters, of course, and it's important to have some opinions at the ready to prove you're listening. It would even be clever to disagree mildly on a few issues—and then gain points by giving in graciously. But don't think for a minute that you have a significant role in running this shindig. Even when it comes to the rehearsal dinner, traditionally the responsibility of the groom's parents, you should not make a move without a freely given go-ahead from her (and, by extension, her mother).

Now, before you get all huffy and start demanding equal rights, just think for a moment how fortunate you are that the Big Wedding is—traditionally, culturally, and (who knows?) perhaps even genetically—the bride's show. It is, remember, a logistical nightmare that makes Operation Overlord seem like a casual vacation trip to Europe. The Big Wedding is a lot of plain hard work and requires extraordinary reservoirs of diplomacy, tact, and management skill. So who needs the grief? Shut up, sit back, and count your blessings. Just be sure to get to the church on time.

And look—keep the whole thing in perspective. Remember: The marriage is what it's all about, not the wedding.

POSTSCRIPT: THE SECOND WEDDING

It goes without saying—at least we didn't say anything until now—that the Big Wedding is also the *first* wedding, if for no other reason than that no person in his (or her) right mind would go through such an ordeal twice in a lifetime. So for any man who feels slighted from being left out of the decision-making loop the first time he middle-aisles it, there is one small, albeit bitter-sweet, consolation: He can always look forward to the Second Wedding.

That's because the Second Wedding is a whole new ballgame. A major difference is that all decisions will be made jointly by the bride and groom (assuming, of course, that the Wedding is the Second for both). Because both of you, now wary, battle-scarred veterans, must be sensitive to each other's old wounds if this event is to come off at all. The Second will almost certainly be a smaller, more personal affair than the Big, and much more likely to be an expression of your personalities than just a reflection of prevailing social practice. Consequently, there will be far more flexibility and opportunity for innovation in the ceremony itself. And probably a lot more fun.

One happily married couple we know first met at a Sunday morning volleyball game in New York City's Central Park. Each had been married previously in a Big Wedding. When, after a whirlwind courtship of some six years, they decided to tie the knot, they rented an old school bus, stocked it with champagne and a tape deck, picked up 30 friends from around the city, took a drive down Fifth Avenue listening to their favorite tunes, and meandered back through the streets of Manhattan to Central Park, where, on a crisp, sunny November day, they were married—on the exact site of their first meeting.

Wouldn't it be great if the Big Wedding could be more like the Second Wedding?

WEEKEND GUEST

"To offer hospitality, or to accept it, is but an instinct which man has acquired in the long course of his self-development. Lions do not ask one another to their lairs, nor do birds keep open nest."

The next time you accept an invitation for a weekend with friends in their country home, ski lodge, or beach house, it would be well to reflect on this observation Max Beerbohm made in a famous essay entitled "Hosts and Guests." And before you conclude that this is a natural enough act not to require a second thought, ask yourself: How often do you drop by the same friends' primary residence back in the city on a Tuesday evening and then stay on for a two-day visit? What might seem at first blush a golden chance for a free mini-vacation can turn into a 48-hour nightmare unless certain basic rules of behavior are observed.

Be on time. Elsewhere (see PUNCTUALITY) we put punctuality right up there with cleanliness as a virtue, and in no instance is this truer than with a weekend visit. Never say, "I'll get there sometime after noon on Friday," unless you're virtually a family member and have the key to your hosts' house. Vagueness about your arrival could tie people up for hours. Say instead, "I'll get there between two and three," and call ahead if heavy traffic, car trouble, a plane/train delay, or just a late start threatens your ETA.

Establish your departure time up front. Maybe your hosts won't fear that you'll turn into "The Man who Came to Dinner," but it will help them plan the rest of their weekend if you let them know exactly when you will be leaving. And in setting the time, think early rather than late. Better to plan a Sunday noon departure and allow yourself to be persuaded to stay over until Monday if everyone is having a good time than to count on the longer stay right out of the box. There's nothing longer than Sunday afternoon in the country when it's pouring rain and the long hike you'd all counted on has been washed out. When isolated and left to their own devices, people can get ugly; witness Jack Nicholson in *The Shining*.

You can't leave just because it's raining. A corollary to the rule about departing on time is that you can't—or shouldn't—bug out just because the weather goes sour. It's tempting, if you arrive at your friends' beach house on Friday afternoon and a storm front settles in Friday evening, to remember a Saturday lunch date that you just can't break and so be on the road back home before breakfast. But you can't, not unless you want your hosts to think that you accepted their invitation in the first place only for the opportunity to soak up rays rather than to bask in the pleasure of their company. Accept fate—and the fact that a rainy weekend at the beach is a perfect time to start *War and Peace*.

Pitch in. A good weekend guest makes his own bed, washes dishes, takes out the garbage, and stands ready to accept even more complex chores (unless your hosts are particularly well-heeled, in which case your toughest job is staying out of the servants' way). Be wary, though, of hosts who are renovating their country place and see weekend guests as a natural source of cheap labor, unless your idea of fun is helping insulate the west wing of someone else's house or chopping enough kindling to last the winter.

Have a game plan. It's enough that your hosts are providing free food and shelter; don't expect them to organize your every waking minute for you. Shortly after you arrive, lay out a few things that you'd like to do—go for a long walk in the woods, explore the antique shops in the next town, pick apples at a nearby orchard, or get up early to go fishing—and see how those plans fit into the agenda your hosts have outlined. A little planning and accommodation on both sides will minimize misunderstanding and disappointment.

Togetherness kills. A thoughtful guest knows the value of making himself scarce. However close you and your hosts might be, odds are you don't customarily spend 12 to 14 straight hours together. Keep that in mind when allocating your time as their weekend guest. If you don't take the initiative to go off somewhere by yourself, they might feel obliged to be doing something with you all the time, and by Sunday night your friendship could be history.

Bring provisions. We're not talking flour and sugar here, but something festive. A couple of bottles of good wine may be a cliché, but few are the homes where they wouldn't be welcome. Don't bring anything that requires cooking unless you've checked in advance with your hosts and are prepared to do it yourself.

Send a gift. You want to be asked back, don't you? Even if you don't, this is one of those times when a gift is definitely called for. Select something particularly appropriate and send it along with a thank-you note within a week after your visit (see BREAD-AND-BUTTER GIFTS and THANK YOU). No need to be extravagant, but do try to pick a gift—probably for the house—that will make your hosts think of you and all the fun you had together every time they see it.

WHO PAYS?

Most males of a certain age have fading but chilling memories of times in their youth when romance and bankruptcy became intertwined. For many, the occasion was high school graduation, when a week of parties and events designed to launch them into technical adulthood required shelling out huge sums of money—for their fun and their girlfriends' as well. No matter that she was graduating, too, or that her daddy was twice as rich as yours. The boy paid. Next question.

But that was in the bad old days. In modern times, if the first date was your idea, you pay. If it was hers, she does. Of course, it gets a little trickier after that.

When two consenting adults with roughly the same middle-class incomes get together socially more than three times, it's patently absurd for one of the two to be stuck with all the restaurant tabs and theater tickets all the time. (And if either has an after-tax income in six figures, it's time to turn the page.) It's an acceptable tribute to custom for the man to cover date expenses at the outset, but once you decide you like each other, chances are she'll say, "May I?" and you'll answer, "If you'd like," and your relationship will be launched, with no more fuss than that, on the righteous path of fiscal sanity.

Let simple equity and common sense be your guide. If she makes twice your salary (don't be so crude as to ask—there are ways to tell), there's no reason why she shouldn't pay for two movie dates to your one. And vice versa. Vacations and weekend trips, split fifty-fifty. Special, out-of-the-ordinary surprises are, of course, always at the exclusive expense of the surpriser, never the surprisee.

Be sure to talk about it if things get out of balance. What's the use of the Communicate Imperative that governs relations between man and woman these days if it's not employed to make certain everyone pays his—and her—fair share?

And remember: There's no such thing as a free lunch—unless she has a generous expense account.

WINE

With all the hocus-pocus spoken and written about wine, the really amazing thing is that some of it actually makes sense—at least to those people who feel like making a study of it. If you're one of those people, you don't need us to give you any tips about how to buy, serve, and drink wine. But if you're just getting started, you've come to the right place.

Serving wine at home is a lot more fun than buying it in fancy restaurants, and not just because you don't have to shell out twice the retail price, either. In your own dining room you can relax and experiment a little, even conduct modest tastings if you've a mind to. You'll probably want to invest in a little equipment before you have company over to sip. The well-stocked glass cabinet has red-wine glasses (medium stems, large, well-rounded bowls), white-wine glasses (long stems, smaller round bowls), and tulip- or flute-shaped champagne glasses. If you want just one glass, start with a red-wine glass with a medium-size bowl—sometimes called the all-purpose wineglass. It will do just fine for white as well.

Next you'll need a reliable corkscrew, one that won't make you look like a complete jerk when the time comes to open the wine. As usual, simplicity is all; the one we like is a bartender's corkscrew with a lever. And then you'll need a simple decanter and some cheesecloth if you're planning to serve old port or red wines old enough to have thrown sediment.

Perhaps the most helpful of all wine miscellany you can keep close by are a wallet-sized vintage chart (it tells you which were the good years, and it's perfectly okay to refer to it at liquor stores and restaurants) and a copy of *Hugh Johnson's Pocket Encyclopedia of Wine*. It's little (that is, *portable*), fact-packed, and relatively undaunting.

Almost as good as having Hugh Johnson as your buddy is making friends with someone who works in a good liquor store. Ask his advice and follow it. If he gives you a bum steer, find another friend.

A basic wine "cellar" might include a case of recent vintage Beaujolais, perfect with pizza, spaghetti, meat loaf, hamburgers, or any casual meal. With fish and seafood take your pick of three recent vintage wines: California Johannisberg Riesling, Italian Verdicchio, or French Muscadet. If you're serving meat, try Chianti Classico, Cabernet Sauvignon, or a moderately priced Bordeaux from a good year (1982 is the best recent year). Chicken is nicely complemented by a Chardonnay from a reliable California producer (Mirassou or Beaulieu, for example). To top it all off, one of the nicest things you can do for yourself or your company is to keep a case of champagne around. Think French and Brut, but forget about vintage. You really can't taste it.

Zoo

Yes, it's a zoo out there, but nowhere is it written—at least not in these pages—that you have to behave like an animal. Good form is not some deep, complicated mystery. All that's required to master it is a genuine regard for the feelings of others and a normal measure of common sense. Bring both to bear on the choices you make and you'll never break an important rule of etiquette that didn't have it coming.

ABOUT THE AUTHORS

Glen Waggoner is a senior writer for *Esquire* magazine, a co-author of *Baseball by the Rules,* and the editor of *Rotisserie League Baseball.* He lives in New York.

Kathleen Moloney, a New York free-lance writer, has written books about health and ventriloquism. She is also a co-author of *Baseball by the Rules.*